Fracture and Fatigue Characterisation of Cortical Bone Tissue

Fracture and Fatigue Characterisation of Cortical Bone Tissue is a key guide to bone fracture and fatigue, focusing on quasi-static and fatigue-fracture characterisation of cortical bone tissue. Discussing the fundamental aspects of fracture mechanics and fatigue, which are applicable to many orthotropic materials, this book examines novel, cutting-edge approaches to analyse and model bone fracture and fatigue.

As the population ages across the globe, bone fracture and fatigue has become a fundamental part of mechanical and biomedical engineering research. Beginning with a thorough description of fracture mechanics and fatigue, the book describes non-linear fracture mechanics under quasi-static and fatigue analyses. It goes on to present a cohesive zone modelling method which is appropriate for mode I, mode II and mixed-mode I+II loading. Presenting the latest research, this book describes cutting-edge fracture tests, new methods for data reduction purposes and numerical models based on cohesive zone modelling. This book is key to aiding both students and professionals in applying fundamental theories and methods to cortical bone tissue.

The book will be of interest to students and professionals working in mechanical engineering and biomedical engineering, including work on quasi-static fracture, fracture under fatigue loading, artificial bones and fracture mechanisms.

Fracture and Fatigue Characterisation of Cortical Bone Tissue

Marcelo F. S. F. de Moura and Nuno Dourado

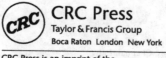

CRC Press
Taylor & Francis Group
Boca Raton London New York

CRC Press is an imprint of the
Taylor & Francis Group, an **informa** business

Designed cover image: Marcelo de Moura

First edition published 2025
by CRC Press
2385 NW Executive Center Drive, Suite 320, Boca Raton FL 33431

and by CRC Press
4 Park Square, Milton Park, Abingdon, Oxon, OX14 4RN

CRC Press is an imprint of Taylor & Francis Group, LLC

© 2025 Marcelo F. S. F. de Moura and Nuno Dourado

ISBN: 978-1-032-45031-5 (hbk)
ISBN: 978-1-032-45032-2 (pbk)
ISBN: 978-1-003-37508-1 (ebk)

DOI: 10.1201/9781003375081

Typeset in Nemilov
by Deanta Global Publishing Services, Chennai, India

Contents

Preface

Bone fractures are common traumas resulting from accidental loading, fatigue, exercise practising, ageing, diseases or pharmaceutical treatments. Hence, they can be viewed as a relevant public health concern resulting in morbidity and mortality, leading to significant economic costs. Damage and fracture of bone reduce the load-bearing capacity of the skeleton and are the origins of serious problems such as injury, loss of flexibility and life quality, collectively leading to health, economic and social problems. In this context, new clinical methodologies and techniques should be developed to identify bone properties associated with its fracture. Consequently, it becomes important to understand the fracture mechanisms of cortical bone tissue, aiming to treat bone traumas and improve the design of artificial bone grafts and implants. Fracture mechanics-based approach is an appropriate method to address this issue. According to this methodology, the material contains an inherent defect and the objective is to verify whether the conditions of its propagation are satisfied. Fracture toughness is the mechanical property that describes the resistance to crack initiation and propagation.

Bones are submitted to fatigue loading during daily life activities. Fatigue is characterised by progressive and localised damage resulting from cyclic loading that occurs below the elastic limit of the material. It raises when the local stresses are high enough to initiate a crack and to promote its propagation until final failure. In this context, the fatigue/fracture behaviour of cortical bone is a relevant topic of research.

The contents of this book include new fracture tests applied to bone, new methods for data reduction purposes and new numerical models based on cohesive zone modelling which proved to be appropriate to mimic damage initiation and propagation in cortical bone tissue. Full descriptions of the fundamentals of fracture mechanics and fatigue are exposed in this book. Non-linear fracture mechanics approaches dedicated to quasi-static and fatigue/fracture analyses are described. Therefore, cohesive zone modelling appropriate for both types of loading is presented. Quasi-static and fatigue/fracture characterisations of cortical bovine bone were performed throughout this book, namely:

- Mode I loading, considering the double cantilever beam test;
- Mode II loading, using the end-notched flexure and the end-loaded split test;
- Mixed-mode I+II loading, employing the single-leg bending and the mixed-mode bending tests.

These tasks provided the identification of the energetic-based criterion for quasi-static loading, as well as the evolution of the Paris law coefficients as a function of the mode mixity for fatigue loading. These laws are crucial for a comprehensive description of damage mechanics of bone under static or dynamic loading.

Several applications of the methodologies exposed all over this book are presented in the last chapter. The analysed cases involve the immobilisation of bone tissue considering different types of fractures.

The aim of this book is to encourage the application of fundamental theories and methods in the context of clinical methodologies and techniques regarding fracture and fatigue loading of cortical bone tissue.

Acknowledgements

The authors thank the Portuguese Foundation for Science and Technology for supporting the work here presented through the projects "Fracture behaviour of cortical bone tissue" (PTDC/EME-PME/71273/2006), "Fracture behaviour of cortical bone under mixed-mode I+II loading" (PTDC/EME-PME/119093/2010) and "Development of an innovative composite system for comminuted bone fracture stabilization" (PTDC/EME-SIS/28225/2017).

The authors would also like to thank Professors Fábio Pereira and José Morais from the University of Trás-os-Montes e Alto Douro (UTAD), Portugal, for their advices, ideas and participation in the generality of the topics. They would also like to highlight and express their gratitude to Professors José Xavier and Maria Isabel Dias for their invaluable contribution to the experimental work. All the students who took part in the research projects are also warmly recognised, namely Teresa Campos.

About the Authors

Marcelo F. S. F. de Moura is Full Professor at the Mechanical Engineering Department of the Faculty of Engineering of the University of Porto, Portugal. His research interests are focused on the mechanical and fracture behaviour of aniso-tropic materials (composites, wood and bone) and adhesive bonding. Numerical simulation of fracture and fatigue using cohesive zone modelling is a prominent research topic. He is the author/co-author of 199 research papers in international scientific journals (h-index = 46 in Scopus considering independent citations) and 3 books; he has participated in 33 research projects, being the leader of 10 of them, and has supervised 15 PhD students (4 ongoing).

Nuno Dourado is Associate Professor at the Mechanical Department of the School of Engineering of the University of Minho in Guimarães, Portugal. His research interests are focused on the fracture characterisation of quasi-brittle materials (wood, concrete and bone tissue) and cohesive zone modelling of these materials' behaviour. The characterisation of the viscoelastic response of bio-logical materials is a recent topic of research. He has authored/co-authored 85 research papers (h-index = 20 in Scopus considering independent citations) and 1 book, has participated in 11 scientific projects, being the leader of 2 of them, and has supervised/co-supervised 49 MSc thesis and 7 PhD students (3 ongoing).

1 Introduction

An adult human body contains more than 200 individual bones. Bones and connective tissues, including muscles and joints, constitute the skeletal system. Bones are strong enough to deal with body weight during daily activities, although they are very light. These characteristics (light and stiff) result from an internal structure similar to a honeycomb. Stiffness and strength are important features of the skeleton to support the body structurally; to ensure body shape functions; for the protection of many vital internal soft tissues (such as heart and lungs) against external loads; for bone marrow support; and for fixation of tendons (in origins and insertions) to connect bones to muscular groups, which is essential to locomotion. They also constitute the body's largest reservoir of mineral ions, particularly calcium, magnesium and phosphorus. Bones are essentially constituted by a soft structure composed of the protein collagen, the mineral calcium phosphate that hardens the soft framework, giving rise to bones' stiffness and strength, and water. They are essentially living cells embedded in a mineral-based organic matrix known as the extracellular matrix. This extracellular matrix is composed of organic components (30–35%), with mostly type I collagen (90% of the organic matrix), inorganic components (65–70%), including hydroxyapatite, and other salts, such as calcium carbonate and phosphate. The organic matrix impregnated by inorganic hydroxyapatite crystals enables bone tissue to withstand high tensile forces (due to the organic matrix) and compression forces (due to the hydroxyapatite crystals). The combination of organic and mineral phases gives rise to the unique biomechanical properties of bone tissue. The organic collagen influences bone elasticity, ductility, viscoelasticity and toughness (i.e., the amount of energy needed to cause a fracture). Alterations of collagen properties can influence the mechanical properties of bone making it more brittle, i.e., increase its fracture susceptibility. On the other hand, mineral content predominantly contributes to bone stiffness and strength. Mechanical properties of bone, like its strength and toughness, result from the mechanical properties of these two phases (organic and inorganic) along with their hierarchical disposition [Liu et al., 2016].

There are two different types of bone tissues according to their structural organisation, the cortical and the cancellous bone. Although they have similar compositions (i.e., they are made up of the same cells and the same matrix elements), they reveal quite different internal structural arrangements and porosity levels, giving rise to remarkably different mechanical properties and functions [Clarke, 2008]. The main characteristics of these types of bones can be summarised as follows:

- Compact or cortical bone is responsible for nearly 80% of skeletal mass; it is dense and solid and constitutes the hard external part of the bone, forming the protective layer around the internal cavity containing the

DOI: 10.1201/9781003375081-1

yellow bone marrow; it is extremely strong and mostly responsible for bearing the mechanical loading as a result of its high resistance to bending and torsion; it also contains a complex network of holes and microscopic channels for blood vessels and nerves.

- Cancellous or spongy bone is softer, weaker and more flexible than compact bone being located inside it; it is very porous and constituted by a lattice-like matrix network of tiny pieces of bone called trabeculae; it is highly vascularised and contains red bone marrow; it fulfils essentially a metabolic function, although it also participates in the biomechanical role in specific sites such as the vertebrae, with great resistance to compressive loads; it is essentially found at the ends of the long bones (the epiphyses), being bounded by the cortical bone.

Bone and connective tissues are very important constituents of the skeletal system, playing significant biomechanical and metabolic functions in vertebrate animals. Bone tissue is the main constituent of the skeletal system, differing from the connective tissue in both stiffness and strength. These physical features result from the existence of inorganic salts that are impregnated within the bone matrix (i.e., water and soft organic materials), which is formed by collagen fibres, diverse non-collagenous proteins and minerals. Minerals in bone tissue are important sources of ions, mostly calcium, contributing to regularise the composition of the extracellular fluid. Bone tissue is also a remarkable self-repairing material, able to locally change its mass, configuration and mechanical properties, as a consequence of intense physical activity, without damaging or causing pain. It is also a very important site for haematopoiesis[1] and endocrine regulation.[2]

From the mechanical response point of view, bone tissue behaves as an orthotropic material, since its elastic properties vary with direction (longitudinal, radial, tangential) and are also heterogeneous, in that there is a field of properties along the bone.

1.1 BONE COMPOSITION

Bone tissue is a living active tissue that is constantly being remodelled. It is constituted by cells embedded in a highly mineralised organic matrix formed by organic and inorganic compounds. The organic phase is formed by collagen[3] (mainly type I),[4] glycoproteins, proteoglycans and sialoproteins [Palmer et al., 2008], while the inorganic is made up of nanofibres, hydroxyapatite (~60%),[5] a naturally occurring mineral form of calcium apatite, and whitlockite,[6] an unusual magnesium-rich calcium phosphate phase whose size can range from 10 to 50 nm (in woven bone[7]) and 20 to 50 nm (in lamellar bone[8]) [Kaplan et al., 1994] deposited along the collagen fibrils. The mineralised matrix gives this tissue an extreme hardness, allowing it to perform important sustaining and protective functions. In turn, the collagen matrix provides it with a certain malleability, giving it some extension and flexion possibilities.

1.1.1 THE ROLE OF COLLAGEN

Collagen, the most prevalent component of the extracellular matrix,[9] has a hierarchical organisation over several length scales [Hillgärtner et al., 2018] (Figure 1.1). This component, representing more than 90% of the organic matrix [Tzaphlidou, 2008], is made of densely packed rod-like mineralised macroscopic fibres and networks that result from an aggregation process of individual triple helices[10] (protocollagen strands), forming tropocollagen molecules (i.e., monomer or "collagen molecule") in a hierarchical manner [Shoulders and Raines, 2009], whose stacking process leads to the construction of fine collagen fibrils (diameter 20–500 nm) (Figure 1.1). The development of those fibrils (fibrillogenesis) starts with a single protocollagen strand (~300 nm long; diameter ≤ 0.8 nm) constituted by parallel chains of amino acids, containing a triple helical segment with N- and C-terminals.[11] Following this process, several enzymes (P4H, P3H, lysyl hydroxylase and protein disulphide isomerase) undergo the modification of certain amino acid residues[12] and folding[13] of three protocollagen strands (≈ 300 nm long) into a triplet helix (trimeric procollagen molecules or procollagen triple helix), which is stabilised by disulphide bridges at the C-telopeptide (i.e., chain terminal). Each of these triple helices (Figure 1.1) is constituted of parallel chains of amino acids (triple-stranded or trimeric procollagen molecules) of the same length (two with the same amino acid compositions, while one with a different one) [Currey, 2002].

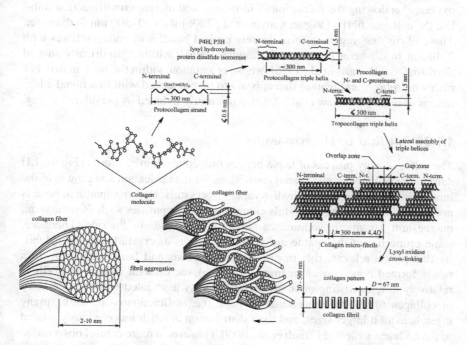

FIGURE 1.1 Hierarchical self-assembly of fibril-forming collagen type I [Shoulders et al., 2009; Banerjee and Azevedo, 2017].

They are held together by interchain hydrogen bonds, in a left-handed extended polyproline II-type helical conformation (a protein-type structure), which coil about each other with a one-residue stagger between adjacent chains to form a right-handed triple helix [Shoulders and Raines, 2009]. These triple helices form procollagen molecules (triple helix), extending from the N-terminus to the C-terminus (N- and C-telopeptides) (<300 nm in length and 1.5 nm in diameter), which have been secreted to the outside of cells and transformed into tropocollagen molecules [Liu et al., 2019], after the site-directed and restrictive cleavage of biological enzymes [Gelse et al., 2003]. Procollagen triple helix thus formed does not have the ability to undergo further self-assembly until proteinases[14] cut off a large fragment of propeptide domains at both ends. The residual folded structure is then referred to as tropocollagen triple helix, measuring on average <300 nm and 1–2 nm in diameter. Tropocollagen triple helix self-assembly takes place in a linear head-to-tail arrangement,[15] with the N- and C-telopeptides appearing each other also laterally (i.e., lateral assembly of triple helices) to make up a quasi-hexagonal unit cell containing five tropocollagen monomers as the basis of the collagen fibril [Bozec et al., 2007]. Arrangements of this type are required on an extraordinary scale to form collagen fibrils at a structural dimension. The formed three-dimensional staggered array of fibrils reveals periodic bands (with period D = 67 nm)[16] between adjacent tropocollagen chains (banding patterns). Subsequent to fibril assembly, telopeptides are covalently cross-linked[17] with the aid of lysyl oxidase,[18] endowing the formation of immature and mature crosslinks that stabilise the collagen fibrils [Viguet-Carrin et al., 2006] with 20–500 nm in diameter. These fibrils[19] aggregate to form densely packed bundles of collagen fibres with 2–10 nm in diameter [Stecco and Hammer, 2015], within cylindrically shaped fibril surfaces [Landis et al., 1996], whose orientation within the bone matrix is a micro-morphological feature that appears to be associated with functional adaptations of bone [Warshaw et al., 2017], particularly induced by prevalent loading.

1.1.2 THE ROLE OF HYDROXYAPATITE

The self-assembly process of triple helices into collagen microfibrils (Figure 1.1) defines the framework and spatial restrictions for the nucleation and growth of the inorganic phase, particularly hydroxyapatite[20] crystals. Hydroxyapatite in bone is not pure, since the apatite crystals contain several impurities such as potassium, magnesium, strontium, sodium, carbonate and chloride or fluoride. Therefore, some properties of the apatite are affected, such as its crystallinity and solubility that play a relevant role in mineral homeostasis and bone adaptation. In a newly formed bone (woven or immature bone), the mineral content in fibrils is relatively low, consisting of small crystals closely associated with the geometry of collagen fibrils. In a more mature bone (i.e., differentiated or adult), many crystals exhibit larger sizes, and their distribution is much less obviously related to the collagen structure [Traub et al., 1989]. However, a more careful observation of those structures reveals that their plate-like crystals are preferentially associated with gaped zones of the collagen fibrils[21] (Figure 1.1), with some crystals at least extending into the overlap regions (~27 nm; Landis et al., 1996). This configuration is believed to be due to the confined space in which the crystals are allowed to grow, which makes them much shorter and thinner than the rod-like apatite crystals of tooth enamel [Traub et al., 1989]. Bone tissue is thus referred to as a platelet-reinforced fibril nanocomposite that contains parallel plate-like hydroxyapatite crystals with their c-axes[22] aligned with the long axis of the fibril (Figure 1.2) [Weiner and Wagner, 1998]. This physical characteristic allows bones to take advantage of the higher strength and stiffness offered by mineral crystals disposed along longitudinal axes.

The process of bone mineralisation is crucial to defining bone hardness and strength. An improper functioning of the mineralisation process leads to

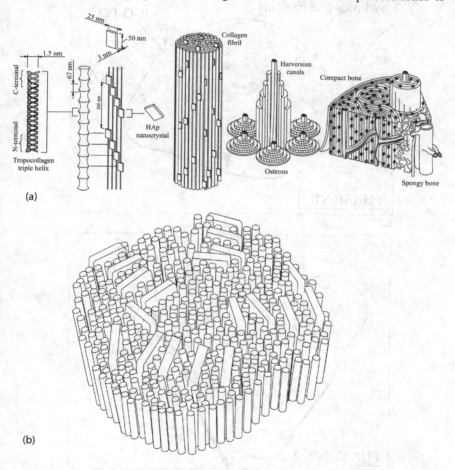

FIGURE 1.2 Scheme showing (a) the hierarchical organisation of bone from mesoscale to macroscale [Landis et al., 1996] and (b) the illustration of the lateral packing of mineral crystals in the collagen matrix. Thin apatite platelets are aligned nearly parallel within the stacks. The crystals are typically about 3 nm thick, 25 nm wide and 50 nm high.

insufficient or excessive mineralisation with adverse consequences on the bone tissue quality causing bone diseases. Bone biomineralisation process acts via a so-called matrix vesicle-mediated mineralisation mechanism,[23] according to which matrix vesicles[24] are secreted by the outer membranes of bone-forming osteoblasts[25] and related cells in a biphasic phenomenon [Anderson, 1995]. Hence, the first phase is characterised by the nucleation of crystals of minerals within matrix vesicles (Figure 1.3a). In this stage, the calcium concentration increases in the intravesicular region due to its affinity for lipids and calcium-binding proteins

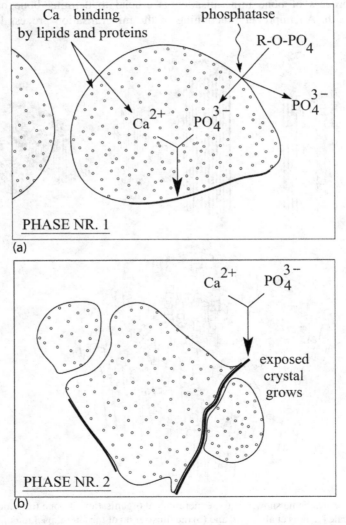

FIGURE 1.3   (a) Mineralisation in matrix vesicles during phase 1; (b) exposure of pre-formed apatite crystals to extravesicular fluid during phase 2 [Anderson, 1995].

contained in the interior of the vesicle[26] membrane. A local increase in phosphate (PO_4) in the vicinity of that membrane is induced on ester phosphate of matrix or vesicle fluid, by phosphatase[27] at the vesicle membrane. The initial deposition of $CaPO_4$ near the membrane is raised by the ionic product $Ca^{2+} + PO_4^{3-}$. The second phase starts when newly formed apatite crystals penetrate the vesicle membrane, exposing minerals to extracellular fluid (Figure 1.3b). From this phase, the growth rate of minerals depends on extracellular conditions such as the concentration of ionic PO_4^{3-} or Ca^{2+} within the extracellular environment (EE), its pH, and the existence of molecules controlling the growth of crystals like anionic proteoglycans [Campo and Romano, 1986; Dziewaitkowski and Majznerski, 1985], and/or calcium-binding non-collagenous matrix protein. This phase is characterised by a slow and gradual maturation of the bone mineral component, an increase in the number of crystals and/or in crystal sizes, and an improvement in the perfection of the crystal arrangement [Boivin, 2007]. This secondary mineralisation is responsible for a progressive increase of the mineral content in the bone matrix.

During the biomineralisation process, the concentration of mineral phase in bone shows a pronounced variation, ranging from low to intermediate and full mineralisation [Fratzl et al., 2004]. Effectively, the independent crystal nucleating and growing deposition are gathered to form a rather continuous, cylindrically shaped streak of minerals along a fibril (Figure 1.4), which extend from a narrow tip (tapered ends of deposition) containing minor and infrequent crystals, to wider regions disposing larger and more numerous and/or more densely packed crystals [Landis et al., 1996]. Some larger crystals extend in length beyond a single period,[28] while a few are laterally interconnected. Regardless of mineral concentration, and despite the scientific debate, most studies describe hydroxyapatite as plate-like crystals [He et al., 2003] of irregular shape (30–50 nm in length; 20–25 nm in width and 1.5–4 nm in thickness) depending on the study [Palmer et al., 2008] (Figure 1.4). The wide range of sizes of hydroxyapatite has to do with the location where the observations have been made, namely within or between the collagen fibrils, and the degree of bone differentiation. Bone mineralisation is a dynamic and continuous process that relies on the correct balance between bone resorption by osteoclasts[29] and bone deposition by osteoblasts.

1.1.3 THE ROLE OF NON-COLLAGENOUS PROTEINS

Non-collagenous proteins form approximately 10% of the organic bone matrix, playing an important role in the regulation of both the mineral nucleation and growth (apatite deposition) in bone biomineralisation processes [He et al., 2003]. Bone sialoprotein, osteonectin, osteopontin and osteocalcin are the most important proteins that form this non-collagenous group.

Bone sialoprotein is one of the major extracellular matrix proteins of the bone and belongs to the small integrin-binding ligand N-linked glycoprotein (SIBLING) family. Bone sialoprotein is a phosphoprotein including large parts of poly(glutamic acids) and the Arg-Gly-Asp (RGD) integrin-binding sequence at its carboxy terminus. This protein is considered physiologically important for

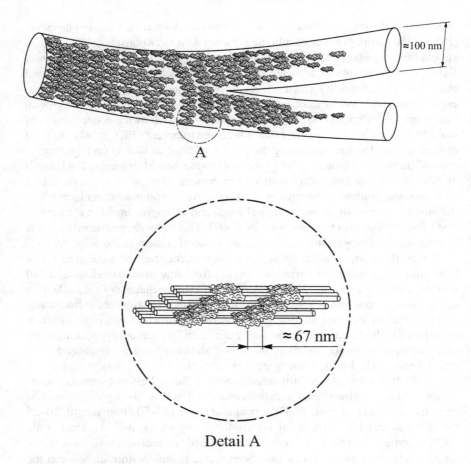

A

Detail A

FIGURE 1.4 Illustration of a fibril constituted by two aggregated segments showing the coherence of collagen segments and alignment of mineral particles tapered ends [Landis et al., 1996].

hydroxyapatite nucleation, cell attachment and collagen binding [Kruger et al., 2014].

Osteonectin is an acidic extracellular matrix glycoprotein responsible for calcium binding and it is produced by osteoblasts during bone formation. Osteonectin regulates the adhesion of osteoblasts and platelets to their extracellular matrix. It plays an important role in the bone mineralisation onset, in the stimulation of the mineral crystal formation, in the cell–matrix interactions and in the collagen binding [Villarreal et al., 1989].

Osteopontin also belongs to the small integrin-binding ligand N-linked glycoproteins (SIBLINGs) family and is one of the major non-collagenous structural proteins in the extracellular matrix of mineralised tissue such as bone [Kruger et al., 2014]. Osteopontin is produced by cells involved in bone morphogenesis such as preosteoblasts, osteoblasts, osteoclasts, osteocytes, odontoblasts and hypertrophic chondrocytes. During bone remodelling, osteopontin contributes to linking osteoclasts to the mineral matrix of bone and plays a relevant role in bone immunoregulation and inflammation.

Osteocalcin is the most abundant non-collagenous protein of the bone matrix (15%) and it is synthesised by the osteoblasts [Boskey et al., 2013]. Osteocalcin is a specific and sensitive biomarker of the bone formation process, since it is present in bone tissue and increases during skeletal growth. In bone, osteocalcin is bound to hydroxyapatite and is released during bone formation and following resorption by osteoclasts. This hydroxyapatite-binding function of osteocalcin contributes to bone mineralisation.

1.1.4 THE ROLE OF BONE CELLS

Four types of bone cells (osteoprogenitor cells, osteoblasts, osteocytes and osteoclasts) assure the bone tissue homeostasis [Brown et al., 2020], i.e., a relatively stable state of equilibrium between bone tissue and interdependent elements of the organism.

Osteoprogenitors are stem mesenchymal cells located in the bone marrow that have the ability to differentiate and proliferate into more specialised bone cells [Vanputte et al., 2020]. Bone marrow is a complex spongy tissue located inside of some bones and its cells are precursors of bone remodelling of cells. In particular, osteoprogenitor cells have the ability to differentiate into osteoblasts, the main cell type constituting bone tissue. Hence, they can be viewed as precursors of osteoblasts and osteocytes and they play an important role in bone repair and growth.

Osteoblasts are osteogenic cells (i.e., bone-producing cells) deriving from mesenchymal stem cells (osteoprogenitor cells) by means of bone extracellular matrix and biochemical signalling [Brown et al., 2020]. Osteoblasts are responsible for the production of collagen type I and non-collagenous proteins, such as osteocalcin, osteopontin and osteonectin [Lacroix, 2019]. Moreover, they produce regulatory and growth factors responsible for bone cell activation, differentiation and growth. Osteoblasts also produce unmineralised osteoid matrix and its subsequent mineralisation leading to a calcification matrix, thus contributing to bone matrix formation. Hence, the osteoblasts are responsible for forming new bone (ossification or osteogenesis) by adding up on the surface of a previously existing layer of bone [Vanputte et al. 2020]. Normally, osteoblasts differentiate into osteocytes through a sequence of maturational stages resulting in the osteocyte. When this process does not take place, osteoblasts undertake apoptosis, i.e., the death of cells that occurs as a normal and controlled part of an organism's growth or development [Brown et al., 2020; Lacroix, 2019].

Osteoclasts are irregularly shaped giant cells (15–20 μm or more) resulting from haematopoietic (monocyte/macrophage – two types of white blood cells) lineage stem cells found in the bone marrow. They are essential in the local removal of bone matrix (resorption of bone) during its growth by secreting hydrochloric acid and during remodelling of osteons and bone surfaces [Brown et al., 2020]. Osteoblasts and osteoclasts play a major and coordinated role in bone modelling, a process that dictates bone change in its structure in response to mechanical and physiological stimuli. Moreover, these bone cells are relevant in injured bone remodelling characterised by continuous and dynamic equilibrium bone resorption and formation allowing it to preserve its functional integrity [Kohli et al., 2018; Uda et al., 2017].

Osteocytes are mature (i.e., terminally differentiated) and the most abundant type of bone cells (90–95% of bone cells) and have a lifespan of up to 25 years [Vanputte et al., 2020]. Osteocytes are located within the bone matrix occupying a fluid-filled space within their lacunae (small spaces between the layers of lamellae) and are sandwiched between adjacent lamellae [Vanputte et al., 2020]. They have an oblong shape and are interconnected by long dendritic through a network of channels (canaliculi) that allows the nutrients to pass through, which is crucial for the osteocyte life and, consequently, for the bone matrix life. This interconnecting arrangement is relevant regarding the mechanosensation and mechanotransduction mechanisms [Rosa et al., 2015]. Mechanosensation consists of the capacity of the osteocyte being sensible to mechanical stimuli that act on the bone. Mechanical stresses, such as those resulting from the action of gravity or muscular activity, are examples of stimuli (static and dynamic). Mechanotransduction can be viewed as the conversion of an external mechanical load into a biochemical cellular response. In other words, the transduction mechanism can be considered as a process by which certain cells (receptor cells) detect or "feel" certain mechanical signals (applied forces or tensions) generating a cellular response of biochemical nature directed to the target cells (effector cells). In fact, osteocytes respond to direct mechanical deformation resulting from bone matrix strain, shear stress owing to fluid flow [Kameo et al., 2022], electric fields induced by stress-generated flowing potentials [Mak and Zhang, 2001] and hydrostatic pressure [Scheiner et al., 2015]. This information is then transmitted to the surface cells that subsequently activate the bone tissue remodelling processes, whenever they are needed [Bonewald et al., 2008; Henriksen et al., 2009].

Bone lining cells result from osteoblasts that do not differentiate into osteocytes and do not suffer apoptosis. When these old osteoblasts finish filling a cavity, they become flattened and elongated cells at the surface of the bone. By covering the bone surface, the main activities of lining cells consist of the preservation of the bone fluids and the fluxes of ions between the bone fluid and interstitial fluid for mineral homeostasis, and the alterations inherent to the natural bone remodelling cycle. They are responsible for the control of calcium exchanges into and out of the bone and they create special proteins that activate the osteoclasts. They also regulate bone remodelling by promoting haematopoietic stem cell differentiation into osteoclasts and favouring communication with osteocytes located inside the bone matrix. In addition, they are responsible for the elimination of the non-mineralised collagen layer from the bone surface before remodelling and subsequent deposition of a new layer of collagen [Brown et al., 2020].

The osteoblasts, osteocytes, osteoclasts and bone lining cells are present on bone surfaces and they play a crucial role in the remodelling process necessary to preserve bone functionality. Hence, bone remodelling occurs in the internal and central surfaces of the osteon and consists of a mechanism of replacement, or reconstruction, of areas of bone tissue in order to preserve its integrity, optimise its function and prevent its degradation. Bone remodelling is essential, aiming to maintain calcium homeostasis to replace hypermineralised tissue with tougher one and to restore damaged bone due to the propagation of microfractures. This process involves an articulation between the resorption of bone promoted by osteoclasts on a particular surface, followed by a stage of bone formation by osteoblasts. The bone state at each moment results from the equilibrium between these two processes. They are particularly useful in bone remodelling in the recovery process after bone fractures and in preventing future bone fractures by recovering microdamage resulting from daily activities. In fact, bone tissue can suffer and accumulate structural fatigue damage (microcracks and damage caused by continued use, i.e., fatigue loading). However, bone tissue has the ability to detect and localise the extent of damage, as well as efficient mechanisms to remove it, restoring the initial state, that is, it has an intrinsic ability to self-repair. This constant responsiveness of bone tissue is achieved essentially through the remodelling processes. In the normal adult skeleton, there is a balance between bone formation and resorption, thus being a permanent dynamic process during all life.

1.1.5 BONE ARCHITECTURE

The cortical (or compact) and trabecular (or cancellous) bones have different structural arrangements at the microscale, although they are identical at the nanoscale. At the macroscale, the most noticeable difference between cortical and trabecular bones lies in the porosity and, consequently, in the density. While cortical bone porosity does not exceed 5%, that of the trabecular exceeds 50%. Since the resistance of bone to compressive loads is proportional to its squared density, the elastic modulus and strength of cortical bone are substantially higher than the trabecular one. On the other hand, trabecular bone presents a higher surface area per unit volume when compared to cortical bone, meaning that its cells are more easily affected by the cells of marrow. Therefore, trabecular bone reveals superior metabolic and remodelling capacities with a consequent faster response to mechanical, chemical and hormonal stimuli.

Cortical and trabecular bone can be divided into two types of bones according to the arrangement of the collagen fibrils: woven and lamellar. Woven (or fibrous or primary) is juvenile bone formed during skeleton growth or in the course of healing of bone tissues after any bone damage event. It results from the rapid production of osteoid by osteoblasts and is characterised by a random disposition of collagen fibres and disorderly calcification, which occurs in irregularly distributed patches. Woven bone is highly mineralised and it is often quite porous at the micron level [Currey, 2002]. This type of bone lays down quickly (more than 4 μm per day), but it is weak. Woven bone is replaced in the normal skeleton by mature lamellar bone after completion of growth, or after any bone damage event in a healing process. Lamellar (or second-ary) bone is the main type of bone in an adult normal skeleton, being more organised and lower mineralised than woven bone. It forms much more slowly (<1 µm per day) than woven bone, it is stronger than woven bone and it is characterised by a regular parallel alignment of collagen fibres. It is arranged in sheets (lamellae), which can be parallel to each other or arranged in a precise concentric form. Lamellar bone is formed by apposition on a pre-existing relatively flat surface to place the collagen fibres in parallel or concentric layers [Royce et al., 2003].

1.1.5.1 Cortical Bone

At the microscale, cortical long bones are essentially constituted of osteons (or Haversian system), which are lamellae cylindrical structures [Farokhi et al., 2018; Vanputte et al., 2020]. The lamellae are layers of compact mineral matrix that surround the Haversian canals (Figure 1.5) in a concentric ring disposition (Figure 1.6). They produce red and yellow bone marrow and they connect the lacunae to the central canal. Osteons are considered the basic structural unit of bone and constitute approximately 70% of cortical bone volume. Each one (Figure 1.2a) contains 10–30 lamellae (each about 5 µm thick), disposed concen-trically around the neurovascular central canal (or Haversian canal), where the blood vessels, nerves and cells are present. Each bone lamella has an orientation approximately perpendicular to the adjacent lamella in order to provide greater

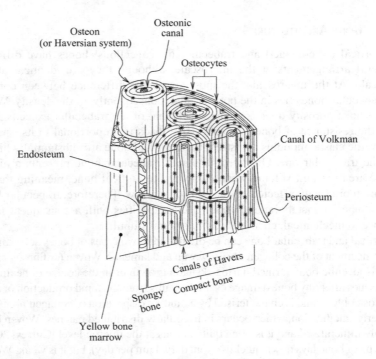

FIGURE 1.5 Schematic representation of bone internal microstructure.

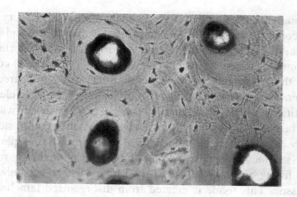

FIGURE 1.6 Optical micrograph showing the morphology of the transverse cross-section of cortical lamellar bone.

resistance to crack propagation. Some oblong spaces called lacunae arise between the layers of lamellae, in which bone cells (osteocytes) are located. The osteon has a diameter of about 10–500 micrometres and a length varying from several millimetres to around one centimetre. Additionally, in the direction transversal to the osteon axis, there are intercommunicating systems (canaliculi, lacunae and Volkmann's canals) connecting the Haversian canals with each other and with the external bone surface (periosteum). They establish a network between the different central channels of the osteons transferring blood vessels from the periosteum into the Haversian canals. These Volkmann's tiny canals contain blood vessels and nerve fibres, and their principal function is to transport nourishing and nutrient elements to osteons [Vanputte et al., 2020]. This bone internal architecture based on the dense network of canals assures appropriate vascularity of bone cells, which is fundamental for bone living and its renewal.

Osteons are cylindrical structures aligned parallel to the long axis of the bone containing a mineral matrix and living osteocytes located in lacunae and connected by canaliculi, which transport blood. They are surrounded by a quite thin layer (thickness of <5 μm) known as the cement line, which is assumed to be the interface between the osteons and the extraosteonal bone matrix. Burr et al. [1988] suggest that the cement line is a poorly mineralised viscous interface, which may contain sulphated mucosubstances. This composition gives rise to a relatively ductile interface with the surrounding mineralised bone matrix. This mismatch stiffness property enhances poor osteon–matrix bonding defining a region prone to crack initiation and slow crack growth in compact bone. This suggests that the cement line can be regarded as a more compliant and weak interface compared to the adjacent bone tissue. Its interfacial properties are relevant to the definition of the failure properties of bone tissue as is the case of the bone fracture toughness. Some authors [Carter and Hayes, 1977; Jepsen et al., 1999] identified experimental evidence of cement line involvement in the failure process of bone tissue such as fatigue or damage in cortical bone. Dong et al. [2000] performed osteon pushout tests with controlled constant displacement rate employing a microtesting machine. Although they verified that these tests are very sensitive to experimental conditions such as supporting hole size, punch size and shape of the selected osteon, they concluded that the cement line is a weak interface between bone tissue lamellae. In a more recent study, Skedros et al. [2005] contested the statement that the osteon cement line is poorly mineralised compared to the surrounding mineralised bone matrix, using qualitative backscattered electron imaging and quantitative energy-dispersive X-ray spectroscopy, each with relatively lower-energy beams. Alternatively, they suggest that the term "osteon reversal region" is more appropriate than "cement line" to describe the complex composite interface that is formed after the reversal of bone resorption during remodelling.

The tissue filling the gaps between the primary osteons is known as interstitial bone tissue. This tissue is created from disorganised lamellar fragments (interstitial lamellae) between intact osteons. The inner side and the outside of the compact bone tissue are filled by inner and outer circumferential lamellae, respectively, running around the circumference of the bone.

1.1.5.2   Trabecular Bone

Trabecular (or cancellous) bone corresponds to 20% of the bone mass in the normal and healthy adult skeleton. The cancellous bone consists primarily of lamellae, arranged in a less organised lattice-like network of matrix spikes, called trabeculae (Figure 1.7). The trabecula is constituted by a three-dimensional mesh of plates and thin rods giving rise to a very porous type of bone. In fact, most

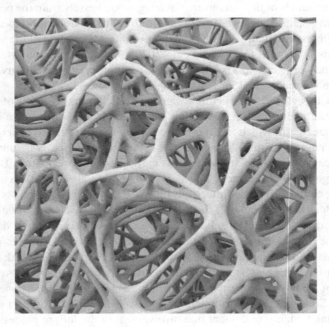

FIGURE 1.7   Optical micrograph of the morphology of the transverse cross-section of a trabecular bone. In: Public Domain Pictures (https://stock.adobe.com/).

trabeculae are thin (in the order of 50–400 μm) and interspersed with large bone spaces (in the order of 500–1500 μm) filled with red bone marrow [Morgan et al., 2013; Shore et al., 2012]. Thin trabeculae are composed of many lamellae, mostly parallel to each other, delimiting wide intercommunicating cavities occupied, in living bone, by red bone marrow. Osteocytes are located in lacunae sandwiched between adjacent lamellae. The trabeculae are organised in the form of a three-dimensional network, always following the lines of the mechanical loading. This type of disposition gives the cancellous bone an optimal resistance to the loads transmitted by the articular surfaces.

The basic structural unit in trabecular bone is the hemiosteon or trabecular packet (approximately 50 μm in thickness and 600 μm long), which is organised similarly to the osteon, but does not contain vascular channels (the Haversian system) (Figure 1.5). In the hemiosteons, lamellae are disposed longitudinally along the trabeculae, i.e., they follow the same shape as the trabecular surface, most of which are concave toward the marrow, in contrast to concentric disposal observed in compact bone osteons. Like in cortical bone, interstitial bone is created from disorganised lamellae between hemiosteons and lacunae. In addition, the small cavities hosting the osteocytes are also found in trabecular bone.

The internal bone architecture and structure arrangement and therefore its mechanical properties are influenced by applied mechanical loading through adaptive sensitive mechanisms, for both cortical and trabecular bones. Consequently, bone mechanical properties depend on several aspects that modify bone microstructure, loading direction and loading mode. The most relevant are the bone anatomic site, its spatial positioning within the long bones, diseases (e.g., osteoporosis, which is a multifactorial disorder associated with loss of bone mass and structure, in which a deterioration of bone strength leads to an increase in bone fragility and a higher fracture risk) and age. These two last are responsible for altering the balance between bone loss and gain giving rise to alterations in the skeleton health. In fact, they increase resorption, resulting in an imbalance of bone remodelling leading to bone loss [Shore et al., 2012; Morgan et al., 2013; Rosa et al., 2015]. In a healthy skeleton, the bone remodelling process preserves the equilibrium between total bone formation and resorption, constantly removing older bone and replacing it with new bone.

1.2 BONE AT THE MACROSCALE

Individual bones and connective tissues joining them constitute the vertebrae skeleton. Bones are hard and stiff, which are fundamental to maintain the shape of the body, to protect the soft tissues and to permit the locomotion transmitting muscular contraction loads from different parts of the body. On the other hand, the connective tissues that include muscles, tendons, fat, and cartilage are softer and more flexible than bone.

At the macroscale, the typical human long bones (i.e., bones that are longer and narrow, as is the case of the humerus, femur and tibia) are complex structures that are composed of cortical and trabecular bone, periosteum, endosteum and articular cartilage (Figure 1.8).

The cortical bone is the exterior wall of all bones and carries out the vital supporting and protecting functions of the skeleton. In long bones, it covers the trabecular bone of the epiphyses, metaphysis and diaphysis (surrounding the medullary cavity). It constitutes the majority of the bone mass (around 80%) in the body and it is 80–90% mineralised. Therefore, cortical bone is a compact and dense structure surrounding the trabecular bone and bone marrow. The mechanical elastic properties of cortical bone (e.g., Young's modulus and strength) are much higher than the ones of the trabecular bone.

Morphologically, long bones (e.g., femur or tibia) are divided into the epiphysis (distal and proximal), metaphysis and diaphysis (Figure 1.8). The epiphyses are the two prominent irregular extremities of the bone, denominated proximal and distal epiphyses depending on its relative position in the body. They consist of cancellous bone surrounded by compact bone (sometimes covered by articular cartilage). The epiphyses are connected to the diaphysis by two conical regions called metaphyses (intermediate zones). The metaphyses are also constituted by cancellous bone surrounded by compact bone and they are known as growth plate (in the proximal region) and fused growth plate (throughout the distal region). The diaphysis is a central cylindrical shaft with regular shape made up of compact bone tissue, with a central medullary cavity filled with bone marrow and some trabecular bone tissue elements. The shape of long bones is intrinsically

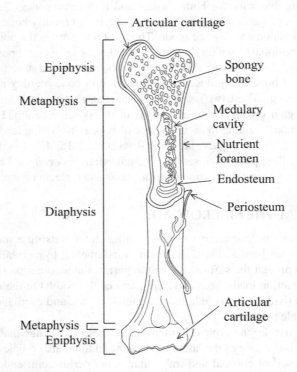

FIGURE 1.8 Typical structure of a long bone.

associated with mechanical loading to which they are submitted. In corpulent and heavy animals, the epiphyses are bigger relative to their diaphysis, comparatively to slender animals. As the epiphyses within the joint region are covered by a film of cartilage (known as articular cartilage), these regions have to have larger areas to transmit the same loads of the diaphyseal region.

The periosteum and the endosteum cover externally and internally the diaphysis area, respectivelly. The periosteum covers all bone tissue surfaces, except the epiphyseal articular cartilage zones, the subcapsular areas and the tendon and ligament insertion zones. It is made up of a tough outer fibrous layer and a thin inner osteogenic layer. The endosteum covers the walls of the bone cavities that contain the bone marrow. It lines the outside of the trabeculae and the wall of the Haversian and Volkmann's canals.

1.3   SUMMARY

Bone tissue is the main constituent of the skeletal system and can be viewed as an outstanding biological material with the particular capacity to build very resistant structures that grow, remodel and repair themselves. In fact, despite its apparently inert appearance, bone is a living active tissue. It is also a highly dynamic structure, which is constantly remodelled throughout the body's life in order to maintain its mechanical properties and capacity. Essentially, bone is constituted by a cellular component and an extracellular matrix composed of a mineral phase (mainly hydroxyapatite), an organic phase (mainly collagen) and water. The mineral phase is mostly responsible for stiffness and strength, while the organic phase and water play an essential role in viscoelasticity and toughness (resistance to fracture).

From the structural point of view, bone can be classified as trabecular and cortical. Trabecular bone is quite porous, soft and flexible, contains the red bone marrow and plays a crucial role in vascularisation and metabolic functions. Cortical bone is dense, hard, stiff and strong, being essentially responsible for the protection of soft tissues and for bearing the mechanical loading induced by normal daily activities of the human body.

The main objective of this book is to perform thorough analyses regarding the fracture behaviour of the cortical bone tissue, taking into consideration its relevant role in the protection, supporting and transmission of loads during common quotidian tasks. In effect, bone fractures occur frequently because of accidents, fatigue, diseases and age. Therefore, detailed fracture analysis of cortical bone is quite an important research subject with a significant impact on public health and social-economic relevance.

NOTES

1. A vital function to the continued production of all blood cell lineages.
2. Set of functions ensured by a system of glands that produce hormones, which go directly into the bloodstream, such as the pituitary or thyroid glands.

3. A generic term for proteins forming a characteristic triple helix of three polypeptide chains (groups of amino acids).
4. To date, 28 different types of collagen have been identified in vertebrates [Liu et al., 2019], but the most common one in the human body is the type I collagen molecule [Gautieri et al., 2009].
5. Or hydroxylapatite, with chemical formula: $Ca_5(PO_4)_3OH$.
6. With chemical formula: $Ca_9(MgFe)(PO_4)_6PO_3OH$.
7. Immature or non-differentiated bone.
8. Mature bone.
9. And the most abundant protein on hearth [Buehler and Wong, 2007].
10. Known as α-helices [Parry, 1988].
11. Known as telopeptides. Triple helices have two telopeptides (Fig. 1.2(a)), which may be used as a biomarkers to measure the rate of bone turnover (i.e., bone remodelling process) [Lin et al., 2016]: C-terminal telopeptide or carboxy-terminal collagen crosslinks (known by CTX) and N-terminal telopeptide or amino-terminal collagen crosslinks (known by NTX).
12. When two or more amino acids combine each other to form a peptide (short chain of amino acids), the elements of water are removed. Following this reaction, the remains of each amino acid is called an amino-acid residue.
13. In chemistry, folding is the process by which a molecule assumes its shape or conformation.
14. A breakdown of proteins into smaller polypeptides or single amino acids. This is accomplished by cleaving the peptide bonds within proteins by hydrolysis.
15. Collagen type I is typical fibrillar collagen that consists largely of rectilinear arrays of collagen fibrils [Adachi et al., 1997].
16. Each period includes a gap and an overlap zone.
17. Extracellular process [Tzaphlidou, 2008] of chemically joining molecules by a covalent bond.
18. An extracellular enzyme [Kumari et al., 2017].
19. According to Traub et al. [1989] fibrils were observed to be elongated rather than round in cross-section.
20. Naturally formed hydroxyapatite is not pure, containing impurities such as carbonate (4–6%) [Lowenstam and Weiner, 1989], sodium (0.9%) and magnesium (0.5%) ions [Glimcher, 1998; LeGeros, 1991] as replacement groups in phosphate and hydroxyl sites, resulting in poorly crystalline, calcium-deficient and carbonated HA.
21. Also called "hole zones", which appear to be the site of mineral nucleation (~1.8 nm in diameter; Burger et al., 2008) since crystals seem to grow and proliferate from this area.
22. In crystallography, a symmetrically unique reference vector, oriented vertically by convention, along which no double refraction occurs.
23. An orchestrated sequence of ultrastructural and biochemical events that lead to crystal nucleation and growth.
24. Cellular structures involved in the intracellular transport of proteins and membranes between organelles and in the release of substances to the outside of the cells (authors' note).
25. Large cells responsible for the synthesis and mineralisation of bone during both initial bone formation phases and later in the bone remodelling.
26. Cellular structure involved in the intracellular transport of proteins and membranes between organelles and in the release of substances to the outside of the cells (authors' note).

27. Enzyme that uses water to cleave a phosphoric acid monoester into a phosphate ion and an alcohol (in alkaline phosphatase, pyrophosphatase or adenosine triphosphatase).

28. Those crystals deposition occurs in the channels created by adjacent hole zone regions (gap regions; Fig. 1.1) of the collagen segments. Other crystals are located in the overlap zones as well.

29. Large multinucleated cells (ranging from 5 to 200 nuclei), occupying small depressions on the bone's surface (known by Howship lacunae), responsible for the dissolution and absorption of bone tissue.

2 Bone Mechanical Behaviour

Cortical bone is a load-bearing hard tissue with various functionalities, such as the ones related to protecting the vital organs, supporting the whole body and enabling leverage and movement of the human body. It is a living material, whose composition varies in function of mechanical and physiological environments. Furthermore, it is well known that bone properties alter with age, physical activity, traumas, diseases and the use of pharmacological agents. Fracture resistance of cortical bone is determined from its mineral density and quality, depicted in its hierarchical structure, variation in material properties and accumulation of micro-cracks. In this context, the evaluation of elastic and strength properties of bone tissue is a prerequisite to characterise its mechanical behaviour. In fact, the elastic properties determine the mechanical behaviour of cortical bone during normal daily activities, while the strength ones define its load-bearing capacity and bone fracture risk. Consequently, these properties are essential for the mechanical integrity of bone tissue and they are used in predictive models for bone fracture behaviour, since these models require complete and accurate input of bone tissue properties. In addition, knowledge of elastic properties is essential for prosthesis design providing important insight into the structural demands of long bone shafts in different planes and at different anatomical positions [Hunt et al., 1998].

Bone tissue is a composite material constituted by different phases: mineral, organic and aqueous. The mineral phase is mainly constituted by hydroxyapatite crystals, which are the main contributors to bone's elastic and strength properties [Currey, 1988a; Hernandez et al., 2001]. The organic phase predominantly consists of collagen type I and plays an important role in the viscoelastic [Bowman et al., 1999; Yamashita et al., 2000] and toughness properties of bone [Zioupos et al., 1999; Wang et al., 2000; Morais et al., 2010]. The role of water is also crucial concerning the mechanical behaviour of bone tissue. Water is present in bone in microscopic pores and within the extracellular matrix. It is known that water decreases with age, i.e., with skeletal growth [Jonsson et al., 1985] and with its progressive mineralisation [Robinson et al., 1979]. Moreover, the distribution of water changes during life. In fact, the quantity of water bound to collagen, to mineral and to the free water in the vascular–lacunar–canalicular cavities alters with age. In effect, Kopp et al. [1989] observed that the interaction of water with collagen diminishes with age. Consequently, it is obvious that the distribution of water within bone tissue influences its mechanical behaviour. In fact, dehydration increases bone stiffness and strength, but decreases its toughness [Currey, 1988b; Nyman, et al., 2006; Morais et al., 2010] and viscoelastic properties [Sasaki et al.,

 DOI: 10.1201/9781003375081-2

1995]. Each one of these phases and the alterations suffered for each one during life contribute to the global mechanical behaviour of bone tissue.

Because of its composition, bone tissue is a material with complex hierarchical structure, heterogeneous and anisotropic. In particular, cortical bone has low porosity and its anisotropy is dictated essentially by lamellar and osteonal orientation. Macroscopically, it is often assumed that bone behaves as a "perfect" composite material [Gottesman and Hashin, 1980], i.e., it is supposed that the material does not contain any voids and the matrix is considered homogeneous. However, the composition of bone tissue is more complex than most engineering composites. Cortical bone tissue is constituted by osteons (fibres) embedded within an organic bonding material (matrix). The osteons have a cylindrical shape of about 10–500 μm in diameter oriented roughly parallel to the longitudinal axis of the bone (Figure 2.1). They are considered as an elastic, isotropic and homogeneous material (fibres) reinforcing the isotropic linear viscoelastic matrix. Organic cement lines and interstitial lamellae constitute the matrix embedding the fibres [Rho et al., 1998]. Perfect bonding between fibres and matrix is usually assumed, which is implemented mathematically by means of displacement continuity between these two entities. Following this assumption, cortical bone tissue can be viewed as a cylindrical orthotropic elastic material at the macroscale. In fact, three mutually perpendicular planes of mirror symmetry whose normals define the principal axes of orthotropy (bone directions: L – longitudinal; R – radial; T – tangential) can be identified (Figure 2.1).

There are differences in stiffness and strength between these directions. Reilley and Burstein [1975] performed compression and bending tests on bovine cortical bone tissue and concluded that longitudinal modulus (E_L) is roughly twice

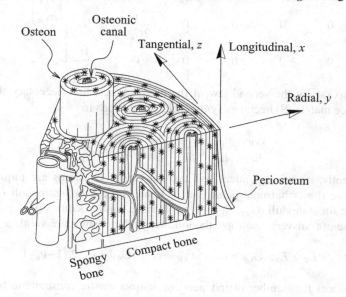

FIGURE 2.1 Orthotropic directions in cortical bone tissue.

the other ones (E_R and E_T). Several authors [Sharir et al., 2008; Guo, 2001] have concluded that Young's modulus is higher in the longitudinal direction when compared to transverse and radial directions, which are similar. Rho et al. [1995] confirmed that transverse and radial moduli are of the same order although they found that $E_T > E_R$ for human cortical femurs. These studies suggest that bone can be viewed as an orthotropic or transversely isotropic material when $E_T \approx E_R$ is assumed. Since transverse isotropy is a particular case of orthotropic constitutive relation, the latter is followed in this book to analyse the elastic behaviour of cortical bone tissue.

Following the orthotropic elasticity theory, the relation between strains (ε) and stresses (σ) can be expressed by the generalised Hooke's law:

$$\varepsilon = \mathbf{S}\sigma \tag{2.1}$$

yielding to

$$
\begin{Bmatrix}
\varepsilon_L \\
\varepsilon_R \\
\varepsilon_T \\
\varepsilon_{RT} \\
\varepsilon_{LT} \\
\varepsilon_{LR}
\end{Bmatrix}
=
\begin{bmatrix}
\dfrac{1}{E_L} & \dfrac{-v_{RL}}{E_R} & \dfrac{-v_{TL}}{E_T} & 0 & 0 & 0 \\[2mm]
\dfrac{-v_{LR}}{E_L} & \dfrac{1}{E_R} & \dfrac{-v_{TR}}{E_T} & 0 & 0 & 0 \\[2mm]
\dfrac{-v_{LT}}{E_L} & \dfrac{-v_{RT}}{E_R} & \dfrac{1}{E_T} & 0 & 0 & 0 \\[2mm]
0 & 0 & 0 & \dfrac{1}{2G_{RT}} & 0 & 0 \\[2mm]
0 & 0 & 0 & 0 & \dfrac{1}{2G_{LT}} & 0 \\[2mm]
0 & 0 & 0 & 0 & 0 & \dfrac{1}{2G_{LR}}
\end{bmatrix}
\begin{Bmatrix}
\sigma_L \\
\sigma_R \\
\sigma_T \\
\sigma_{RT} \\
\sigma_{LT} \\
\sigma_{LR}
\end{Bmatrix}
\tag{2.2}
$$

In order to satisfy the second law of thermodynamics, it is necessary that the compliance matrix ($\mathbf{S}$) becomes symmetric, which leads to

$$\frac{v_{LR}}{E_L} = \frac{v_{RL}}{E_R}, \quad \frac{v_{LT}}{E_L} = \frac{v_{TL}}{E_T}, \quad \frac{v_{RT}}{E_R} = \frac{v_{TR}}{E_T} \tag{2.3}$$

Consequently, nine independent and distinct elastic constants are required to characterise the orthotropic behaviour of bone: three Young's moduli (E_L, E_R, E_T), three shear moduli (G_{RT}, G_{LT}, G_{LR}) and three Poisson's ratios (v_{RT}, v_{LT}, v_{LR}). In the case of transverse isotropy, the following relationships are valid,

$$E_R = E_T; \quad G_{LR} = G_{LT}; \quad v_{LR} = v_{LT}; \quad G_{RT} = E_T/2/(1+v_{RT}) \tag{2.4}$$

which reduces the number of independent distinct elastic constants to be measured to five.

Different laboratorial tests have been applied to estimate the mechanical properties of bone. The most common tests are tensile or compression, three- or four-point bending, torsion, hardness measurement by nanoindentation, ultrasonic continuous wave technique and laser interferometry [Kruzic et al., 2009; Shahar et al., 2007].

Specimens' preparation requires special procedures that depend on the tests to be performed. Long cortical bone specimens are generally dissected from the medial region of tibiae or femurs and immediately cleaned and wrapped in gauze containing a saline solution and frozen at –20°C. Subsequently, the samples are submitted to milling and cutting operations to get the required final dimensions. During these procedures, the endosteal and periosteal tissues are removed and specimens are kept moist using a physiological saline solution. Hydration is also important while cutting and milling to avoid heating the specimens, which would alter the elastic and strength material properties. In the following, the tests and methods frequently employed to obtain the mechanical properties of bone are described in more detail.

2.1 TENSILE AND COMPRESSION TESTS

Tensile tests are used to determine elastic and strength properties in bone. However, one of the most important difficulties intrinsic to the mechanical characterisation of bone regards the specimen size that is possible to get from slabs. Tensile test specimens must be relatively long to provide a useful length allowing representative evaluation of strains. This aspect limits its usefulness when testing cancellous bone or short bones existing in the skeleton. In long cortical bones (e.g., tibiae and femurs), they are used to evaluate the properties along the longitudinal direction (Figure 2.1). The specimen length of bovine bones is usually in the range of 15–40 mm, and it must be carefully machined to assure perfect alignment to induce tensile loading without spurious bending. The cross-sectional squared area at the central region of the specimen (Figure 2.2) should be smaller than the ends, aiming to ensure that strains are occurring essentially in this region [Reilly et al., 1974]. Strains are monitored by means of clip-on extensometers that are attached to the central region of the specimen. The elastic modulus is a proportional constant that establishes the relation between induced stresses (σ_L) and the resulting strains (ε_L). Hence, the longitudinal modulus (E_L) is obtained from the initial slope of the load–displacement curve,

$$E_L = \frac{\Delta P l_1}{\Delta \delta A} \qquad (2.5)$$

where $A = Bh$ stands for the cross-sectional area of the specimen, l_1 is the distance covered by the used extensometer and ΔP and $\Delta \delta$ represent the increment of load and displacement, respectively, between two points located on the initial linear region of the load–displacement curve. The corresponding tensile strength (σ_{uL}) is given by

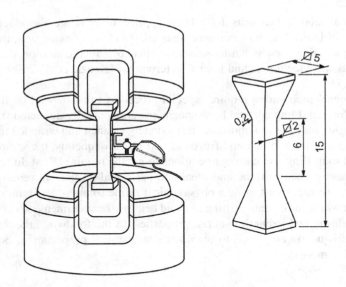

FIGURE 2.2   Geometry of the bone tensile specimen [Reilly et al., 1974].

$$\sigma_{uL} = \frac{P_{max}}{A} \qquad (2.6)$$

where P_{max} is the highest load attained during the test.

Poisson's ratios quantify the lateral deformation resulting from an axial load. They can be measured in tensile tests considering additional extensometers to measure deformation perpendicular (R and/or T directions) to the loading direction,

$$\nu_{Lj} = -\frac{\varepsilon_j}{\varepsilon_L} \; ; \; j = R,T \qquad (2.7)$$

The employment of tensile tests to evaluate Young's moduli in directions R and T is not easy, owing to the limitations on specimens' dimensions possible to get along those directions. Reilly and Burstein [1975] have succeeded in cutting specimens in the RT plane (Figure 2.1) only for bovine bone (the required specimen size precluded this test in human bone), which they considered as a transversely isotropic material. With these specimens, they determined the elastic ($E_R = E_T$ and $\nu_{LR} = \nu_{LT}$) and strength properties ($\sigma_{uR} = \sigma_{uT}$) of bone in the radial and tangential directions.

In contrast, compression tests can be used considering smaller specimens. Shahar et al. [2007] considered small cubes of $2 \times 2 \times 2$ mm^3 of equine cortical bone to perform compression tests. The cubes were cut such that their faces were aligned with the anatomical axes of the bone (Figure 2.3) and loaded along one of the three orthogonal directions (L, R, T). Displacements along and across the loading direction were measured by a non-contact optical-based method using

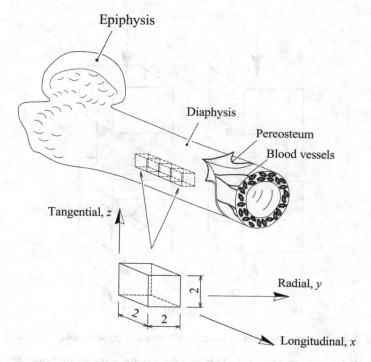

FIGURE 2.3   Cubic specimens harvested from cortical bone (dimensions in mm).

two orthogonally aligned horizontal and vertical speckle pattern-correlation interferometers, which allows for determining the corresponding strains. The three Young's moduli (E_L, E_R, E_T) and three of the six Poisson's ratios of cortical bone were obtained using relations similar to the ones given by Eqs. (2.5) and (2.7). The remaining three Poisson's ratios were obtained by Eq. (2.3).

Compression tests are also frequently used to obtain properties in cancellous bone, owing to difficulties in getting specimens with dimensions compatible with tensile tests. Anyway, it should be noted that compression tests present some difficulties. Specimens must be loaded concentrically between loading platen to minimise spurious effects due to small misalignments (Figure 2.4a) influencing the measured values. The employment of spherically seated loading heads allowing pivoting (Figure 2.4b) assures compressive loading without bending and minimises the influence of misalignment errors. Another aspect that should be considered in compression tests addresses the friction effects between the specimen's loaded faces and loading platens. These friction effects constrain the expansion of the specimen in directions orthogonal to loading one (Poisson's effects) and influence the measured stiffness. Turner and Burr [2001] suggest the employment of petroleum jelly as a lubricant aiming to reduce these unwanted effects.

The referred drawbacks make compression tests less accurate than tensile ones. Anyway, compression tests have an important advantage regarding smaller

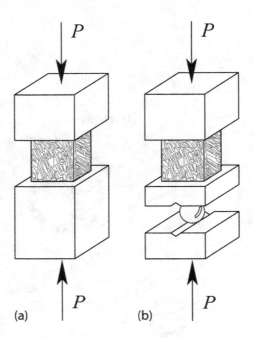

FIGURE 2.4 Compression tests in bone: (a) without and (b) with spherical joint.

specimen dimensions required. This is relevant for cancellous bone, for some bones of the skeleton that do not provide specimens with the length necessary for tensile tests, and for bones that work predominantly under compression *in vivo*, as is the case of vertebrae.

2.2 BENDING TESTS

Bending tests can be used to identify the mechanical properties of cortical long bones. Three-point or four-point bending loading can be employed (Figure 2.5) to estimate the longitudinal modulus and tensile strength.

The three-point bending test is quite simple and consists of the central loading of a simply supported beam (Figure 2.5a). This test has the disadvantage of developing high shear stresses at the mid-section of the bone where loading is applied. The Euler–Bernoulli equation can be used to determine the longitudinal modulus,

$$E_\mathrm{L} = \frac{\Delta P L^3}{6 \Delta \delta I}. \tag{2.8}$$

with L being the specimen length, I the second moment of area of the cross-section of the specimen (i.e., $8Bh^3/12$ for a rectangular section), and ΔP, $\Delta \delta$ the increment of load and deflection at the centre of the specimen, respectively, in the initial linear portion of the load–displacement curve. Owing to the referred shear

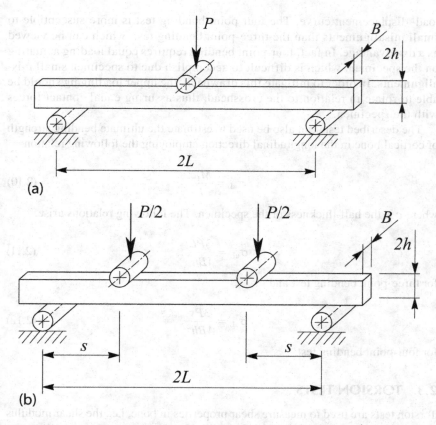

FIGURE 2.5 Schematic representation of (a) three-point bending and (b) four-point bending tests.

effects, the modulus given by Eq. (2.8) is usually called the "apparent" modulus. The agreement between the apparent modulus with the true one increases with the growth of span-to-depth ratio ($L/h \geq 20$ provides good agreement) and Young's versus shear modulus (ratios higher than 14 are advisable). When these conditions are not satisfied, a valuable alternative is the employment of the four-point bending test (Figure 2.5b). This test consists of symmetrically loading a simply supported beam and has the advantage of having a pure bending moment in the central region of the specimen, i.e., between the loading pins. The longitudinal modulus is given by

$$E_{\mathrm{L}} = \frac{\Delta P s^2 (3L - 2s)}{6 \Delta \delta I}. \tag{2.9}$$

with s being the distance between each support and the closest loading point (Figure 2.5b) and ΔP, $\Delta \delta$ the increment of load and deflection at the centre of the loading jig, respectively, in the initial linear portion of the load–displacement curve. The four-point bending test is more susceptible to small misalignments than the three-point bending test, which can be viewed as a disadvantage. In fact, four-point bending requires equal loading actuating on the specimen, which is difficult to accomplish due to specimen small misalignments. In order to mitigate this drawback, the upper loading jig should be able to rotate in relation to the crosshead, thus assuring equal contact forces with the specimen.

The described tests can also be used to estimate the ultimate bending strength of cortical bone in the longitudinal direction employing the following relation:

$$\sigma_{uL} = \frac{M_f c}{I}.$$ (2.10)

where c is the half-thickness of the specimen. The following relations arise,

$$\sigma_{uL} = \frac{3PL}{4Bh^2}.$$ (2.11)

for three-point bending test and

$$\sigma_{uL} = \frac{3Ps}{4Bh^2}.$$ (2.12)

for four-point bending test.

2.3   TORSION TESTS

Torsion tests are used to measure shear properties in bone, i.e., the shear modulus and ultimate shear strength. Specimens with circular, rectangular or hollow sections are the most used in this context (Figure 2.6).

The shear modulus relates the induced shear stress to the resulting shear strain (Eq. 2.2). The following relation can be employed for the shear modulus [Timoshenko et al., 1951] in the longitudinal-transversal or longitudinal-radial plane G_{Li} with $i = $ T, R

$$G_{Li} = \frac{M_t L}{\theta J}.$$ (2.13)

and for the shear strength,

$$\sigma_{uLi} = \frac{M_t c}{J}.$$ (2.14)

being M_t the torsional applied moment, L the specimen length, θ the angle of twist and J the torsional constant that depends on the specimen geometry. For the circular cross-section and hollow specimens, J represents the second polar moment of area of the section (Figure 2.6), respectively,

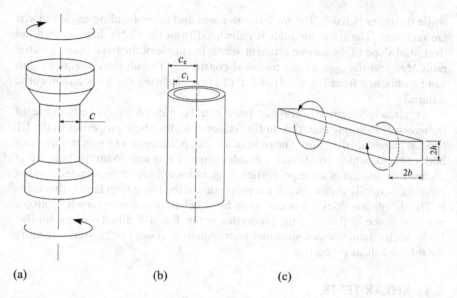

(a)   (b)   (c)

FIGURE 2.6 Specimens used in torsion tests in bone.

$$J = \frac{\pi c^4}{2}; \quad J = \frac{\pi(c_e^4 - c_i^4)}{2}. \tag{2.15}$$

where c, c_e and c_i stand for the radius of the circular and hollow sections. In the case of a rectangular section, the torsional constant J becomes [Timoshenko et al., 1951],

$$J = 16h^3b\left(\frac{1}{3} - \frac{64h}{\pi^5 b} \sum_{i=1,3,5,\ldots}^{\infty} \frac{1}{n^5} \tanh\frac{\pi n b}{2h}\right) \tag{2.16}$$

where h and b (Figure 2.6) are the half-rectangular section dimensions ($b>h$). The ultimate shear stress is given by Timoshenko et al. [1951],

$$\sigma_{uL(T,R)} = \frac{2M_t h}{J}\left(1 - \frac{8}{\pi^2} \sum_{i=1,3,5,\ldots}^{\infty} \frac{1}{n^2 \cosh\frac{\pi n b}{2h}}\right)c. \tag{2.17}$$

The extremities of bone specimens should be firmly embedded in rectangular or cylindrical blocks of a polymer-based material and fixed into the grips of the torsion-loading device. Special care should be dedicated to this task since small misalignments of these blocks relative to the specimen axis can induce spurious bending stresses that affect the results. Moreover, it must be assured that the blocks are really fixed to the bone since any sliding also gives rise to an underestimation of torsional stiffness. The twisting moment is applied to one of the grips while the other is fixed. The torsional moment and corresponding angle of twist are recorded. The shear modulus is calculated from Eq. (2.13), bearing in mind the initial slope of the torsion moment versus the angle of the twist curve, i.e., the ratio M_t/θ and the appropriate torsional constant J. The ultimate shear strength can be obtained from Eq. (2.14) or Eq. (2.17) considering the torsion moment at failure.

As already discussed, cortical bone can be viewed as an orthotropic of transversely isotropic material. In the former case, the shear properties in the LT and LR planes are different. The twist of a bone specimen in a torsion test involves both of them, which constitutes a disadvantage of this test. With the purpose of accurate evaluation of these properties, large ratios b/h are recommended making torsion essentially dependent on the properties of the plane with larger dimension b. This limitation does not occur when bone behaves as a transversely isotropic material, since in this case the properties in the T and R directions are similar. Under such circumstances, specimens with square sections can be used to identify the referred shear properties.

2.4 SHEAR TESTS

Because of the several difficulties inherent to the torsion tests, shear tests can be viewed as a good alternative to measure the shear properties of bone. The main goal of these tests is to induce a state of pure shear loading at the critical section of the specimen from an applied uniaxial loading. The Iosipescu [ASTM standard D5379/D5379M] and Arcan [ASTM standard D7078/D7078M] tests (Figures 2.7a-b) are used in this context for shear characterisation of artificial composites. They are based on rectangular beam specimens of small dimensions with symmetric V-notches (90°) at its centre (Figure 2.8a-b) aiming to create an almost constant shear stress distribution at the critical section. These 90° notches with 3 mm depth [Turner et al., 2001] have fillets to avoid stress concentrations that would induce premature failure of the specimen. These tests are similar to each other in principle and specimen configuration although the loading mode is

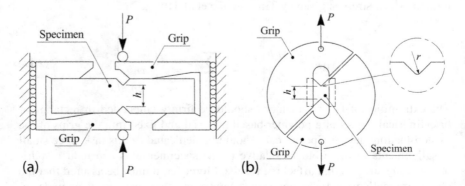

FIGURE 2.7 Schematic representation of the (a) Iosipescu and (b) Arcan tests.

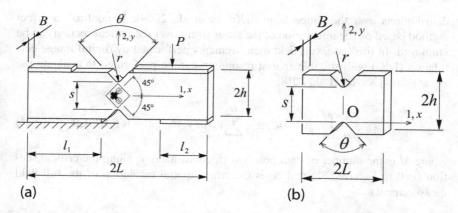

FIGURE 2.8   Schematic representation of the (a) Iosipescu and (b) Arcan specimens.

different. In the Iosipescu test, loading is applied to the specimen thickness faces, while in the Arcan case it is applied to its longitudinal larger faces by tightening it inside the texting fixture (Figure 2.7b). In both, an almost pure shear loading is obtained in the smallest cross-section. The main advantage of these tests in the context of bone shear characterisation is the employment of small specimens (especially in the Arcan case), which makes them appropriate to apply to different planes. Turner et al. [2001] considered $40 \times 10 \times 3$ mm³ specimen dimensions for transverse shear tests with the Iosipescu setup and $10 \times 10 \times 3$ mm³ in the case of Arcan for longitudinal and transverse shear tests. Ultimate shear strengths can be given by

$$\sigma_{u,ij} = \frac{P_u}{A}; \quad ij = RT, LT, LR \tag{2.18}$$

where P_u is the ultimate load and A is the area of the critical section. Shear moduli can be obtained from the elastic domain of the shear–strain curve using the Hooke's law

$$G_{ij} = \frac{\bar{\sigma}_{ij}}{\bar{\varepsilon}_{ij}}; \quad ij = RT, LT, LR \tag{2.19}$$

being $\bar{\sigma}_{ij}$ and $\bar{\varepsilon}_{ij}$ the nominal averaged shear stress and shear strain, respectively. The shear strain is usually measured by means of a strain gauge rosette with two elements oriented at ±45° relative to the longitudinal axis (Figure 2.8a). The shear strain in the material principal axis becomes

$$\bar{\varepsilon}_{ij} = \varepsilon_{45°} - \varepsilon_{-45°}; \quad ij = RT, LT, LR \tag{2.20}$$

However, this procedure requires the determination of numerical correction factors to account for non-uniformities on both shear stress and shear strain distributions over the gauge length [Xavier et al., 2004]. In contrast, a direct method based on the integration of the shear strain over the critical section can be employed. In this case, full-field measurements performed by digital image correlation (DIC) with suitable spatial resolution can be performed to evaluate the shear strain [Xavier et al., 2018],

$$\bar{\varepsilon}_{ij} = \frac{1}{d} \int_0^d \varepsilon_{ij}(0, y)\,dy \cong \frac{1}{d} \sum_{k=1}^{M} \varepsilon_{ij}(0, y_k)\Delta_\varepsilon \;;\; ij = \text{RT,LT,LR} \qquad (2.21)$$

where M is the number of data points with coordinates y_k along the critical section (x=0 in Figure 2.8b) and Δ_ε is the strain spatial resolution of the full-field measurements.

2.5 MECHANICAL TESTS AT THE STRUCTURAL SCALE

The major drawback inherent to the tests described in previous sections is related to the difficulty of specimens' production. In fact, it is very difficult to machine specimens with required dimensions from some bone types (e.g., vertebrae) or from bones of small animals. In these cases, tests on the whole bone can be performed to measure the structural properties of the entire bone. These structural measurements are not directly related to the bone tissue properties since both, material properties and its geometry, contribute to the structural response.

Bending tests (Figure 2.9) are frequently used to test bone at the structural level [Sharir et al., 2008], namely for long bones of small rodents which, owing to their small dimensions, render difficulty in the manufacture of specimens.

In the majority of the published works, the identification of the mechanical properties is based on the Euler–Bernoulli beam theory [Akhter et al., 2004; Bonnet et al., 2007; Sun et al., 2009]. Following this procedure, the bone irregular geometry is assumed to be regular and uniform [Turner and Burr, 1993]. Bone cross-section (Figure 2.10) is usually simulated using an equivalent hollow

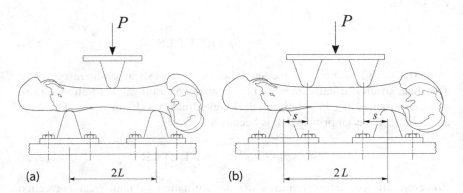

FIGURE 2.9 Schematic representation of the (a) three-point bending and (b) four-point bending tests using entire bone.

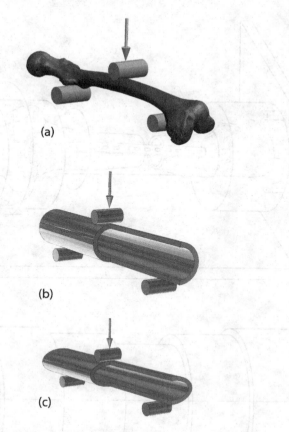

(a)

(b)

(c)

FIGURE 2.10 (a) Realistic; (b) hollow circular and (c) elliptical model to simulate bone at the structural level.

circular [Sharir et al., 2008; Lenthe et al., 2008] or elliptical model [Turner and Burr, 1993]. However, some bones (e.g., the human tibia) have geometries that are not approximately circular nor elliptical and are poorly represented by simple cross-sectional shapes. Moreover, this methodology ignores bone anisotropy and long bones complex geometry, which usually presents discrepancies relative to the assumed approach, thus resulting in erroneous estimations of bone tissue properties [Sharir et al., 2008; Lenthe et al., 2008].

Torsion tests are also applied to bone tissue at the structural scale [Levenston et al., 1994] submitting the whole bone to a shear deformation (Figure 2.11a) aiming to evaluate its structural properties (e.g., torsion moment to failure and torsion moment per angle of twist). Ideally, the strains at the critical region (minimum cross-section) are measured with strain gauges during the torsion test, aiming to determine material properties from the torsion moment. Material properties such as the ultimate shear strength and the average shear modulus can be estimated when detailed knowledge of the bone geometry is available. For example, the assumption of a circular section is a good approximation at the mid-diaphysis

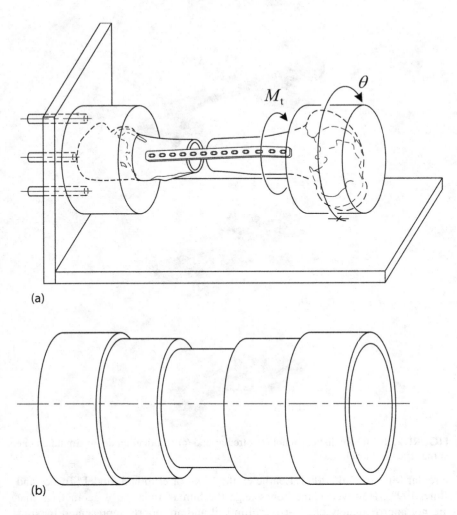

(a)

(b)

FIGURE 2.11   (a) Torsion test applied to entire bone and (b) multi-prismatic model [Levenston et al., 1994].

of the human femur, and it is expected that reasonably accurate estimates can be achieved. Anyway, the employment of constant cross-sectional geometry does not comply with the circumstance that real bones have geometries that vary considerably along the length of the diaphysis, which can lead to inaccurate evaluation of mechanical shear properties. In order to solve this drawback, Levenston et al. [1994] proposed an accurate geometric model incorporating a lengthwise geometric variation of bone cross-sectional geometry. The suggested multi-prismatic model consists of scanning and digitising several cross-sections along the bone in order to simulate the non-prismatic bone as a series of n prismatic segments. An analytical approach applied to the resulting multi-prismatic model (Figure 2.11b) was used to predict the shear elastic modulus. For the particular cases of circular or hollow circular sections, the global bone angle of twist can be written from Eq. (2.13)

$$\theta = \frac{M_t}{G_{Li}} \sum_{j=1}^{n} \frac{L_j}{J_j}. \tag{2.22}$$

where L_j and J_j are the length and the second polar moment of area (Eq. 2.15), respectively, of each segment j. Assuming an odd number of n equally spaced sections ($n \geq 3$), the segment lengths are defined as

$$L_j = \frac{L}{n-1} \begin{cases} 1/2, & j = 1 \\ 1, & j = 2, ..., n-1. \\ 1/2, & j = n \end{cases} \tag{2.23}$$

Combining Eqs. (2.23) and (2.22) yields

$$\theta = \frac{M_t L}{G_{Li}(n+1)} \left[\frac{1}{2} \left(\frac{1}{J_1} + \frac{1}{J_n} \right) + \sum_{j=2}^{n-1} \frac{1}{J_j} \right]. \tag{2.24}$$

An effective second polar moment of area can be defined from Eq. (2.22)

$$J = (n-1) \left[\frac{1}{2} \left(\frac{1}{J_1} + \frac{1}{J_n} \right) + \sum_{j=2}^{n-1} \frac{1}{J_j} \right]^{-1}. \tag{2.25}$$

The effective shear modulus G_{Li} predicted by the multi-prismatic model can now be obtained from Eq. (2.13).

An alternative to estimating the mechanical properties of bone tissue is the application of the inverse methods [Sousa, 2018]. These approaches combine experimental testing with finite element analysis. Computed axial tomography (CAT) with three-dimensional reconstruction software can be employed to define the finite element mesh (Figure 2.12a) used for testing simulation (Figure 2.12b). The procedure consists of an algorithm that performs the segmentation of the CAT images and generates the mesh from them. This segmentation process is particularly advantageous since it allows us to distinguish between cortical and trabecular bone tissues. In contrast, the bone specimen can be sectioned at several locations after testing that are photographed aiming at digital reconstruction of the geometrical model representative of the original bone shape, which is then meshed for finite element analysis (Figure 2.12c).

Subsequently, an optimisation algorithm based on three-dimensional finite element analysis (Figure 2.12b and 2.12c) is applied aiming to reproduce numerically the experimental measured parameters. In the case of elastic moduli, the optimisation procedure is based on the minimisation of the difference between the numerical and experimental initial stiffness directly measured in the load–displacement curve, altering iteratively the design variable (elastic modulus).

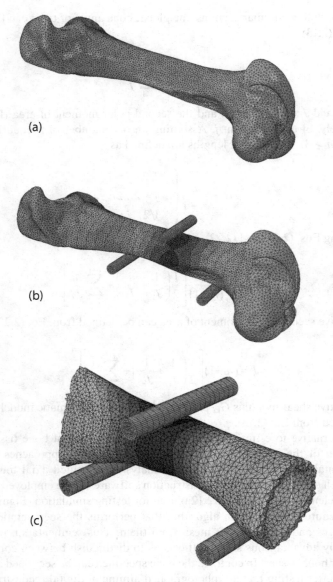

FIGURE 2.12 (a) Finite element mesh generated by CAT; (b) respective numerical displacement field under three-point bending and (c) numerical displacement field under three-point bending with a mesh generated from bone specimen sectioning.

2.6   INDENTATION TESTS

The indentation technique has been employed to determine elastic modulus, strength and hardness of trabecular and cortical bone. This procedure is based on an actuator of high resolution that presses an indenter over the highly polished sample surface, registering the resultant load–displacement relation. The unloading stiffness $dP/d\delta$ (Figure 2.13) is used to estimate the elastic modulus following the relation [Rho et al., 1997],

$$\frac{1-v_b^2}{E_b} = \frac{dP}{d\delta}\sqrt{\frac{\pi}{4A\beta^2}} - \frac{1-v_i^2}{E_i} \tag{2.26}$$

where E_i, E_b and v_i, v_b stand for elastic moduli and Poisson ratios, respectively, of the bone (subscript b) and indenter (subscript i), A is the projected area of the elastic contact [Doerner and Nix, 1986] and β is a factor that depends on the indenter geometry (spherical, cylindrical, conical, pyramidal). The contact area A is given by the optically measured area of the hardness impression. The determination of the bone modulus (E_b) requires the previous knowledge of the bone Poisson's ratio (v_b). Aiming to determine E_b, Rho et al. [1997] assumed $v_b = 0.3$ and performed a sensitivity analysis varying v_b in the range 0.2–0.4. They verified that the values of E_b varied no more than 8%, which makes acceptable the consideration of a typical value for v_b.

Equation (2.26) assumes a homogeneous and isotropic material. Its application to an orthotropic material like bone implies measurements in different directions (L, R, T) to determine the individual elastic constants. A single cubic small

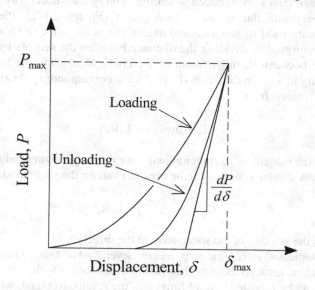

FIGURE 2.13 Experimental evaluation of the unloading stiffness employed in the indentation test to measure the elastic modulus.

specimen allows measuring all of the elastic moduli, which is an advantage of this test.

Indentation tests can also be used in the context of bone strength determination, which can be estimated as the maximum load divided by the cross-sectional area of the indenter. The hardness, H, which physically represents the mean pressure the material can support, is determined from the ratio between the maximum load and the projected area of the contact impression.

Bone is a heterogeneous material whose material properties vary over very small distances as a function of its constituents. In this framework, micro-indentation and nanoindentation tests can be employed to determine the elastic properties of some bone components. These tests require a highly polished specimen surface. Micro-indentation methods provide spatial resolution varying from 30 to 100 μm and nanoindentation applies in the range 1 to 5 μm allowing the measurement of the properties of internal bone constituents and microstructures, like individual bone lamellae, osteons and individual trabeculae [Rho et al., 1997; Zysset, 2009]. Consequently, these methods permit mapping the spatial distribution of superficial mechanical properties of bone with good resolution.

2.7 ACOUSTIC AND ULTRASONIC TESTS

The acoustic and ultrasonic tests are based on the travelling of a normal (speed of sound) or a high-frequency acoustic wave, respectively, through solids. Two types of waves can be generated. The longitudinal ones result when the driving transducer vibrates in the direction of wave propagation (Figure 2.14a). Instead, shear waves are induced when the driving transducer vibrates in the direction perpendicular to wave propagation (Figure 2.14b). Piezoelectric transducers are used to generate and detect waves for velocity measurement, which is performed by dividing the distance between the sensors by the pulse transit time between them [Ashman et al., 1984]. Measuring the longitudinal wave velocity in a given direction (L, R, T), the corresponding elastic modulus can be determined from,

$$E_i = \rho v_{Li}^2 \; ; \; i = \mathrm{L,R,T} \tag{2.27}$$

where v_{Li} is the velocity of the longitudinal wave in the direction i and ρ the material density. A similar equation can be used to evaluate the shear moduli,

$$G_{ij} = \rho v_{Si}^2 \; ; \; i,j = \mathrm{L,R,T} \tag{2.28}$$

where v_{Si} is the velocity of the shear wave in the direction i.

The acoustic and ultrasonic tests present several advantages when compared with mechanical tests. As these methods are non-destructive to the specimen, measurements can be repeated several times and the results averaged, which diminishes the experimental errors. Moreover, one single specimen can be employed

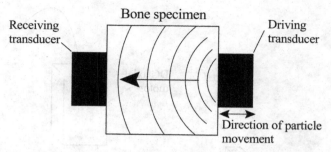

(a)   Longitudinal wave propagation

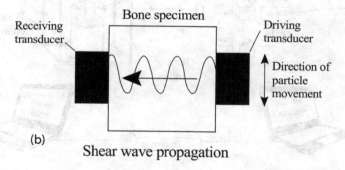

(b)

Shear wave propagation

FIGURE 2.14 Schematic representation of the (a) longitudinal and (b) shear waves' propagation.

to measure the properties in different directions characterising the anisotropy of bone [Hunt et al., 1998]. These methods also require smaller and simpler tests when compared to mechanical test-based procedures. However, these procedures cannot be applied to determine directly the material strength [Turner and Burr, 1993], which is a disadvantage.

2.8   OPTICAL METHODS

Optical methods have several advantages since they allow non-contact measurement of displacements on surfaces of samples subjected to mechanical loading and include the possibility of full-field results. Two main techniques have been employed in the context of bone. The electronic speckle pattern-correlation interferometry (ESPI) [Shahar et al., 2007] allows us to measure displacements directly determined from variations of laser light reflected from samples immersed in water (Figure 2.15). Such measurements can be performed in the elastic region of load–displacement curve, i.e., without damaging the specimen. Another interesting aspect of this technique is the possibility to measure strains along two perpendicular directions (axial and lateral strains) on the specimen surface, which allows the determination of Poisson's ratios from the same experimental data on

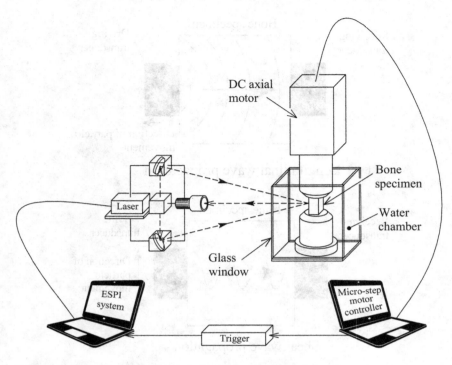

FIGURE 2.15 Schematic representation of the ESPI experimental setup.

exactly the same sample under identical loading conditions. Therefore, the ortho-tropic Young's moduli and Poisson's ratios can be determined from multiple measurements of each sample.

Another technique is the digital image correlation, which is based on the comparison of two speckle patterns obtained before and after loading the specimen, thus providing the displacement that occurred between these two stages. The displacements are measured from two images captured at those stages. With this aim, digital image correlation uses a computer to record the position of the points on the surface before loading and to analyse the changes that occur when the specimen is loaded (Figure 2.16). In bone, the random speckle pattern is created by spraying black ink on the bone surface using an airbrush. The accuracy of the measured displacements is sensible to speckle size in combination with the used pixel subset. Consequently, the choice of a pixel subset should be in agreement with the expected strain field [Lecompte et al., 2006]. Aspects like lack of parallelism between the sensor and the material surface (Figure 2.16), image distortions induced, for example, by a defective lens, noise on the obtained images and others can have a remarkable influence on the image acquisition or pattern quality. These features should be carefully addressed in the experimental work to minimise their influence on the measurements.

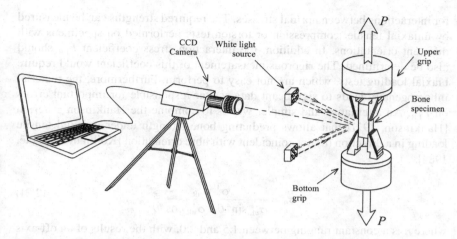

FIGURE 2.16 Schematic representation of the DIC experimental setup.

2.9 STRENGTH FAILURE CRITERIA

As a consequence of the human's daily activities, bone is commonly submitted to multiaxial loading that induces a multiaxial stress state. In this framework, it is advisable to employ multiaxial failure interactive criteria that account for the combined effects of stress or strain components resulting from applied loading. The interactive criteria are based normally on stress quadratic functions, which should be appropriate for orthotropic materials in the case of bone. The Tsai–Wu quadratic criterion [Tsai and Wu, 1971] is one of the most well-known interactive failure criteria. It was initially developed for fibre-reinforced composite materials and it was applied in the context of cortical bone [Hayes and Wright, 1977, Cezayirlioglu et al., 1985, Cowin, 1986]. The general form of the Tsai and Wu tensorial quadratic polynomial criterion used is

$$F_{ij}\sigma_{ij} + F_{ijkl}\sigma_{ij}\sigma_{kl} = 1 \quad ; \quad i,j,k,l = \text{L, R, T} \tag{2.29}$$

where F_{ij} and F_{ijkl} are first-order and second-order strength tensors, respectively, determined experimentally. In the case of orthotropic materials under plane stress in the LR plane, the Tsai–Wu criterion simplifies and yields to

$$\left(\frac{1}{\sigma_{uL}^t} - \frac{1}{\sigma_{uL}^c}\right)\sigma_L + \left(\frac{1}{\sigma_{uR}^t} - \frac{1}{\sigma_{uR}^c}\right)\sigma_R + \frac{\sigma_L^2}{\sigma_{uL}^t\sigma_{uL}^c} + \frac{\sigma_R^2}{\sigma_{uR}^t\sigma_{uR}^c} + 2F_{LR}\sigma_L\sigma_R + \frac{\sigma_{LR}^2}{\sigma_{uLR}^2} = 1 \tag{2.30}$$

The linear terms distinguish tensile from compressive strengths (superscripts "t" and "c", respectively), making this criterion more consistent with the bone's real behaviour. The quadratic terms define an ellipsoid in the stress space and account for interactions between normal stresses. The required strengths can be measured by uniaxial tensile, compression or torsion tests performed on specimens with different orientations. In addition, the interaction stress coefficient F_{LR} should also be determined. The rigorous measurement of this coefficient would require biaxial loading tests, which are not easy to perform. Furthermore, the material inhomogeneity leads to significant data scatter responsible for important errors on F_{LR}. An alternative and simpler way is to combine the Hankinson criterion [Hankinson, 1921] that allows predicting bone strength under uniaxial tensile loading in a direction (θ) not coincident with fibre orientation [Kollman and Coté, 1984],

$$\sigma_\theta = \frac{\sigma_{uL}^t \sigma_{uR}^t}{\sigma_{uL}^t \sin^n \theta + \sigma_{uR}^t \cos^n \theta} \tag{2.31}$$

where n is a constant ranging between 1.5 and 2.0, with the results of an off-axis test [Liu, 1984], which leads to

$$F_{LR} = \frac{1}{2}\left(\frac{1}{\sigma_{uL}^t \sigma_{uR}^c} + \frac{1}{\sigma_{uL}^c \sigma_{uR}^t} - \frac{1}{\sigma_{uLR}^2} \right) \tag{2.32}$$

This procedure satisfies the stability condition

$$F_{LL}F_{RR} - F_{LR}^2 \geq 0 \tag{2.33}$$

that must be fulfilled to guarantee that the criterion (Eq. 2.30) represents a closed ellipsoid. This methodology substitutes the execution of the cumbersome biaxial test by using a simpler off-axis test.

2.10 SUMMARY

The procedures and methods described in this chapter addressing bone strength are generally focused on stress or strain analyses assuming that the material is a continuum media. However, bone is a quite heterogeneous natural biological material having internal defects and presenting drastic variations in its inner structure and its orthotropic properties. These issues make fracture mechanics concepts more reliable than stress or strain-based analyses to deal with bone mechanical behaviour, contributing to a better comprehension of fracture phenomena in cortical bone tissue. The next chapter presents a detailed description of the fundamentals of fracture mechanics theory and the required extensions to account for cortical bone fracture specificities, related to its complex damage mechanisms.

3 Quasi-static Fracture and Fatigue/Fracture Characterisation

Nowadays, bone fractures in the elderly population are a relevant public health concern, since they result in morbidity, mortality and significant economic costs [George and Vashishth, 2006]. Actually, with the increase in life expectancy, bone fracture becomes a significant health problem in older age, due to the alteration in its microstructure and material properties. Bone fractures are common traumas resulting from accidental loading, fatigue, ageing, exercise practicing, diseases or pharmaceutical treatments, all of them leading to skeletal fractures. Damage and fracture of cortical bone reduce the load-bearing capacity of the skeleton and origin serious problems such as injury, loss of flexibility and life quality collectively leading to health, economic and social problems. Generally, bone fracture occurs with more frequency in older age groups suffering from osteoporosis. In this context, it is necessary to develop and implement new methodologies and clinical techniques to identify patients at risk and how to proceed to check and prevent whether action is needed. The lack of these preventive diagnoses inhibits the correct post-fracture assessment, since the initial state is unknown. Nevertheless, stress fracture and trauma cases are also frequent in young active individuals, as is the case of military personnel, athletes and dancers. It is also relevant to assess how different implanted devices, such as screws, nails and wires, and their removal, affect the cortical bone fracture. Consequently, it becomes important to understand the fracture mechanisms of the cortical bone aiming to treat bone traumas and to improve the design of artificial bone graft and implants. For all of these reasons, it becomes evident that fracture characterisation of bone is a crucial research topic with a relevant impact on public health, which justifies its social-economic relevance.

3.1 QUASI-STATIC FRACTURE

Bone is a natural material with an internal heterogeneous microstructure leading to drastic variations in its inner structure, which influences its mechanical behaviour, namely its strength. Examples are the presence of voids, e.g., osteocyte lacunae or Volkmann canals, which mechanically can be viewed as defects. They act as stress concentrators and make difficult accurate predictions of strength owing to their sensitivity to the presence of these singularities. In this framework, stress or strain-based criteria can only give rough approximations to bone strength. In

DOI: 10.1201/9781003375081-3

fact, these criteria assume that the material is free of defects, which is not the case with bone.

An appealing alternative is to employ fracture mechanics concepts. In this method, it is assumed that the material contains an inherent defect and the objective is to verify whether the conditions of its propagation are satisfied. Fracture toughness is the mechanical property that describes the bone resistance to crack initiation and propagation. The determination of the *Resistance*-curve (*R*-curve), which relates the evolution of fracture toughness as a function of the crack length is a crucial feature. This approach relies on non-linear fracture mechanics concepts, in contrast with most of the works based on theories ensuing from linear elastic fracture mechanics to determine fracture toughness. In view of the aforementioned heterogeneous internal microstructure of bone and its complex fracture mechanisms, the suitability of the non-linear fracture mechanics for dealing with bone fracture becomes evident.

3.2 FATIGUE/FRACTURE OF BONE

Fatigue is a phenomenon of progressive weakening of a material when subjected to cyclic loading. It is characterised by progressive and localised damage when the local stresses are high enough to initiate a crack and to promote its propagation until the final fracture. Fatigue can be classified as a type of loading occurring below the elastic limit of the material. Hence, failure due to fatigue occurs in the elastic regime and far from the static limit strength of the material, thus becoming frequent and dangerous. Fatigue loading acts as a cumulative effect that induces material failure after repeated application of stresses, not exceeding the ultimate strength. The term fatigue is based on the concept that a material becomes "tired" and fails at a stress level below the nominal strength of the material. Material mechanical properties (stiffness and strength) degrade over time because of the formation of small cracks within the material microstructure. Three main stages are usually identified during fatigue loading (Figure 3.1): damage onset (Region I), characterised by nucleation of micro-cracks from microstructural defects; these micro-cracks frequently coalesce into a macro-crack that propagates in a stable manner (Region II); final collapse (Region III) is characterised by a sudden increase of damage growth rate leading to final failure. Fatigue design is focused on Region II, aiming to minimise the damage growth rate, thus increasing the life of the structural component. The well-known Paris relation applies to this region, which explains the common designation of "Paris law region" (Figure 3.1).

Fatigue/fracture behaviour of cortical bone tissue is a relevant aspect. In particular, fracture under fatigue loading acquires special relevancy with a remarkable impact on public health owing to population ageing. Bone fatigue occurs under cyclic loading related to normal daily activities, as is the case of walking or running that often initiate and/or promote bone fractures *in vivo*. The formation of micro-cracks in bone is a real, physiological event. Linear micro-cracks in human cortical and trabecular bone have been attributed to *in vivo* fatigue loading, i.e.,

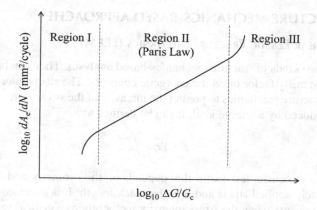

FIGURE 3.1 Typical fatigue behaviour. Bi-logarithmic plot of damage area growth rate as a function of normalised strain energy release rate.

bone fatigue/fracture is generally a result of small cracks that grow with cyclic loading under different loading modes and coalesce into a macro-crack. It should be noted that the natural processes of self-healing, *in vivo*, result in a more favourable fatigue strength than that determined in laboratory tests. This circumstance gives rise to a conservative estimate of fatigue life in the presence of subcritical cracks [Ritchie et al., 2004].

Two different approaches can be employed regarding fatigue analysis: the classical fatigue life determination using the stress versus number of cycles (*S/N*) curves and the fatigue crack propagation (*da/dN*; *a*, crack length; *N*, number of cycles) that allows an easier interpretation for fatigue micro-mechanisms. The traditional fatigue life tests assume that specimens are defect-free when subjected to cyclic loads under different stress values (*S*) to determine the corresponding number of cycles (*N*) leading to failure (*S–N* curves) [Carter and Caler, 1983; Zioupos et al., 1996; Martin, 2003]. However, this type of testing is quite limited regarding the identification of the aspects governing the initiation and propagation of damage during fatigue action [Ritchie et al., 2004]. Cortical bone tissue is a natural material holding micro-defects due to its heterogeneous structure [Carter and Caler, 1983], which means that the fatigue crack propagation phase is predominant. In this context, the application of fracture mechanics concepts emerges as an essential tool to assess bone quality, to improve the diagnoses of fracture risks and to promote the treatment of bone diseases. The awareness of fractures induced by fatigue was relatively recent and adds the concepts of fatigue/fracture as a new study branch of fracture. One of the crucial aspects has to do with the accumulation of fatigue damage throughout life and when it will give rise to a fracture [Acevedo et al., 2018].

In this book, new tests, new procedures for data reduction and new numerical approaches regarding quasi-static fracture and fatigue/fracture behaviour of cortical bone tissue are discussed and proposed.

3.3   FRACTURE MECHANICS-BASED APPROACHES

3.3.1   LINEAR ELASTIC FRACTURE MECHANICS (LEFM)

There are two kinds of fracture mechanics-based analyses. They can be based on
the stress intensity factor or on the energetic concepts. The stress intensity factor
is used in fracture mechanics to predict the intensity of the stress state close to the
crack tip induced by a remote load. It can be defined as

$$K = Y\sigma_R \sqrt{\pi a} \tag{3.1}$$

where Y is a dimensionless factor that depends on the geometry and loading, σ_R
is the remotely applied stress and a is the crack length. It is assumed that crack
propagation occurs when the stress intensity factor attains a critical value

$$K_c = \sigma_u \sqrt{\pi a} \tag{3.2}$$

where σ_u is the material strength. In contrast, an energetic approach based on the
concept of strain energy release rate (G) given by

$$G = \frac{dW}{dA} - \frac{dU}{dA} \tag{3.3}$$

can be employed, where W is the work performed by external forces applied to
the body, U is its internal strain energy and dA is the increase of crack surface.
From Eq. (3.3), it can be settled that G represents the energy released per unit area
when the work performed by external forces becomes higher than the internal
strain energy of the body due to damage occurrence. As a general statement, it
can be affirmed that energetic criteria assume that crack propagation will occur
whenever the strain energy release rate equates to the critical strain energy release
rate (G_c), which is a material property.

Considering a general body with constant thickness B (Figure 3.2) under loading P normal to crack plane, it can be written as

$$W = P\delta \quad ; \quad U = \frac{1}{2}P\delta \tag{3.4}$$

Combining Eqs. (3.3) and (3.4) and using the body compliance $C = \delta/P$ it leads to

$$G = \frac{P^2}{2B}\frac{dC}{da} \tag{3.5}$$

which is known as the Irwin–Kies relation [Irwin and Kies, 1954]. During crack
growth, Eq. (3.5) gives rise to the energy necessary to fracture propagation (G_c)
that is representative of the material fracture behaviour.

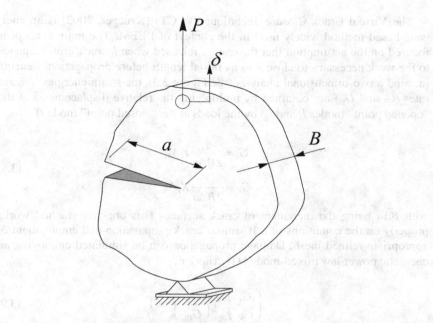

FIGURE 3.2   Cracked body under uniaxial loading.

These two methods are interrelated. In fact, the two fundamental parameters of each one, K and G, are related. Irwin [1957] demonstrated that in plane stress

$$G = \frac{K^2}{E} \tag{3.6}$$

and in plane strain

$$G = \frac{K^2 \left(1 - \upsilon^2\right)}{E} \tag{3.7}$$

where E and υ are the Young's modulus and Poisson's ratio, respectively. These relations also apply to the corresponding critical values (K_c and G_c).

The energetic methods are better suited for heterogeneous materials as is the case of bone. The stress intensity factor is a local parameter evaluating the local stress field close to the crack tip. It works as a scaling factor that describes the alteration of the stress state in the vicinity of the crack tip, being markedly influenced by material heterogeneity. Instead, the energetic criteria are based on global fracture parameters evaluating the energy absorption of all samples during fracture, thus being less sensible to local material variations. Consequently, being a global parameter, G_c is more appropriate than K_c to measure toughness, because K_c can be drastically affected by local variations of the internal material constitution.

The Virtual Crack Closure Technique (VCCT) [Krueger, 2002] is an energetic-based method widely used in the context of LEFM. The main concept is focused on the assumption that the energy released when a crack grows equates to the work necessary to close it to its initial length before propagation. Bearing in mind a two-dimensional analysis (see Figure 3.3), the strain energies' release rates (G_I and G_{II}) are obtained by multiplying the relative displacements at the "opened point" (nodes l_1 and l_2) by the loads at the "closed point" (node i)

$$G_I = \frac{1}{2B\Delta a} Y_i \Delta v_l$$
$$G_{II} = \frac{1}{2B\Delta a} X_i \Delta u_l$$

(3.8)

with $B\Delta a$ being the increment of crack surface. This one-step method works properly on the conditions of self-similar crack propagation and employment of appropriate refined mesh. Damage propagation can be simulated employing an energetic power-law mixed-mode I+II criterion,

$$\left(\frac{G_I}{G_{Ic}}\right)^\alpha + \left(\frac{G_{II}}{G_{IIc}}\right)^\beta = 1$$

(3.9)

with G_{Ic} and G_{IIc} being the fracture energies under modes I and II, respectively, and α, β the mixed-mode fracture parameters determined from experimental testing.

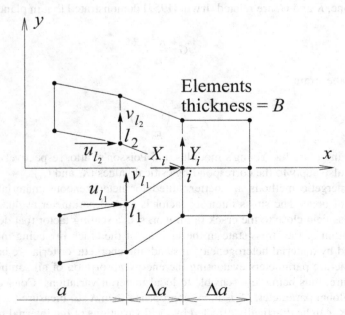

FIGURE 3.3   The Virtual Crack Closure Technique (VCCT).

The elementary assumption of the LEFM is that the damaged zone (the region where several inelastic and dissipative processes take place) in the vicinity of the crack tip it is small and confined. This condition is satisfied in brittle materials but not verified in quasi-brittle materials, as is the case of bone. In fact, the referred damaged zone, usually identified as the fracture process zone (FPZ), reveals a non-negligible size in cortical bone tissue because of its composition and micro-structure. Actually, several toughening mechanisms responsible for a non-negligible dissipation of energy have been identified in the fracture of cortical bone, such as diffuse micro-cracking, crack deflection, osteon pull-out, uncracked ligament bridging and fibre bridging [Zioupos, 1998; Vashishth et al., 2000; Yeni and Norman, 2000; Nalla et al., 2003; Yan et al., 2006]. Commonly, bone fracture starts with the development of very small cracks from microscopic defects. As a result of loading, these small cracks grow and coalesce leading to a propagating macro-crack with the corresponding FPZ, in which the energy dissipation is non-negligible. This fracture mechanism renders inexact the application of the pure LEFM theory in the context of bone fracture characterisation. Furthermore, LEFM always assumes the existence of a crack, thus not being appropriate to predict crack initiation, which constitutes a limitation. Although the former works addressing bone fracture relied on LEFM [Norman et al., 1995; Norman et al., 1996], recent investigations point to the employment of cohesive zone models in this context [Yang et al., 2006; Ural et al., 2006; Morais et al., 2010]. In general, all of these studies emphasised that cohesive zone models are able to capture and predict the behaviour related to bone fracture by representing the physical processes occurring near a propagating crack. In conclusion, these models can be viewed as being non-linear fracture mechanics-based methods, since they are able to account for the energy dissipated in the non-negligible FPZ.

3.3.2 Cohesive Zone Models (CZMs)

Both the stress (or strain) and fracture mechanics-based approaches reveal disadvantages. The strength of materials approaches based on stress (or strain) analyses are useful to identify the most critical points, but they are unable to deal with singularities and reveal important mesh dependency when used in finite element modelling. Fracture mechanics-based approaches rely on the existence of an initial flaw, but in many situations, the identification of the damage initiation locus can be difficult. In order to solve the weaknesses of both methodologies, cohesive zone models (CZMs) combine a stress-based method to identify the critical points prone to damage onset with the fracture mechanics approach to deal with damage growth. Therefore, it is unnecessary to consider an initial defect and mesh dependency complications vanish. The CZM can be integrated in finite element analysis enabling the assessment of the influence of several factors controlling fracture initiation and non-self-similar crack propagation in cortical bone tissue. The typical bone damaging processes are simulated through a softening relationship between stresses and relative displacements between crack faces, thereby mimicking gradual material properties degradation. The softening relationship is implemented in finite element analysis through interface finite elements with null thickness and quite high initial stiffness, and they are positioned at the regions where damage is likely to occur.

In this book, bone fracture under quasi-static and fatigue loading is investigated using CZM. These models provide flexibility and economy in studies and can help to understand underlying mechanisms that might be difficult to discover experimentally, making them very useful complements to experimental studies. They can contribute to a better understanding of how changes in bone tissue quality, especially in the case of the aged and those suffering from bone damaging diseases, affect the onset and propagation of bone fracture.

In this context, two mixed-mode I+II CZMs appropriate for quasi-static and fatigue loading are presented in the following sections.

3.3.2.1   Quasi-static Mixed-Mode I+II CZM

A mixed-mode I+II CZM considering trapezoidal-bilinear softening law (Figure 3.4) appropriate for quasi-static fracture analysis is presented. The softening relationship is established between stresses and relative displacements and intends to mimic damage initiation and propagation in materials. The trapezoidal-bilinear law is appropriate to deal with damage mechanisms in bone, which reveals tough behaviour when hydrated [Morais et al., 2010]. It should be noted that this model is able to be transformed into simpler trapezoidal or triangular cohesive laws, since both are particular cases of the more general trapezoidal-bilinear softening law. In all cases, the cohesive law can be divided into two main parts: the initial linear elastic one up to local strength is attained and, after that, a second one

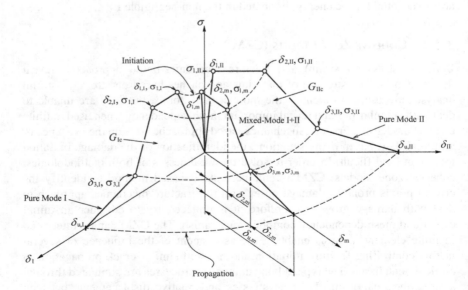

FIGURE 3.4   Trapezoidal with bilinear softening cohesive mixed-mode I+II zone model.

characterised by a softening decrease of the initial stiffness. In the former case, the matrix relation before damage onset becomes

$$\sigma = \mathbf{E}\delta \qquad (3.10)$$

with $\mathbf{E}$ being a diagonal matrix containing the stiffness parameter k, whose value (typically in the range 10^6–10^7 N/mm^3) is selected taking into account two restrictions: low values induce spurious interpenetrations, and quite high values give rise to numerical instabilities [Gonçalves et al, 2000]. After damage onset, the constitutive softening relationship between stresses (σ) and relative displacements (δ) is implemented by means of a damage parameter (d) included in the diagonal matrix $\mathbf{D}$

$$\sigma = (\mathbf{I} - \mathbf{D})\mathbf{E}\delta \qquad (3.11)$$

where $\mathbf{I}$ is the identity matrix. The evolution of the damage parameter between undamaged state ($d=0$) and complete failure ($d=1$) is based on the incremental calculation of energy dissipation during fracture in each integration point. Damage onset under mixed-mode I+II loading (identified by subscript "m") is predicted employing the quadratic stress criterion,

$$\left(\frac{\sigma_{1,m,I}}{\sigma_{1,I}}\right)^2 + \left(\frac{\sigma_{1,m,II}}{\sigma_{1,II}}\right)^2 = 1 \quad \text{if} \quad \sigma_I > 0$$

$$\sigma_{1,m,II} = \sigma_{1,II} \qquad\qquad \text{if} \quad \sigma_I \leq 0 \qquad (3.12)$$

where $\sigma_{1,m,i}$ and $\sigma_{1,i}$ ($i = $ I, II) represent, respectively, the stress components of the mixed-mode I+II loading and the strengths in each pure mode (Figure 3.4).

Combining equations (3.10) and (3.12) for the case $\sigma_I > 0$,

$$\left(\frac{\delta_{1,m,I}}{\delta_{1,I}}\right)^2 + \left(\frac{\delta_{1,m,II}}{\delta_{1,II}}\right)^2 = 1 \qquad (3.13)$$

where $\delta_{1,i}$ and $\delta_{1m,i}$ ($i = $ I, II) are the relative displacements corresponding to damage initiation under pure and mixed-mode I+II loading, respectively (Figure 3.4). Considering a ratio between displacement loading modes,

$$\beta = \frac{\delta_{m,II}}{\delta_{m,I}} \qquad (3.14)$$

and the equivalent current mixed-mode relative displacement

$$\delta_m = \sqrt{\delta_{m,I}^2 + \delta_{m,II}^2} \qquad (3.15)$$

the mixed-mode equivalent relative displacement leading to damage onset can be defined as (Figure 3.4)

$$\delta_{\mathrm{1m}} = \frac{\delta_{1,\mathrm{I}}\delta_{1,\mathrm{II}}\sqrt{1+\beta^2}}{\sqrt{\delta_{1,\mathrm{II}}^2 + \beta^2\delta_{1,\mathrm{I}}^2}} \tag{3.16}$$

After initiation, progressive damage follows the mixed-mode I+II trapezoidal-bilinear softening cohesive law for a given mode ratio (Figures 3.4 and 3.5). The region O-A-B-E in Figure 3.5 represents the energy dissipated in the course of the loading process up to the increment $j-1$ (G_{d}^{j-1}) at a given integration point. Assuming damage progression, the increase of energy in each mode i (i = I, II) for the current increment j is given by

$$\delta G_i^j = \frac{\sigma_i^j + \sigma_i^{j-1}}{2}\left(\delta_i^j - \delta_i^{j-1}\right) \tag{3.17}$$

The total energy dissipated in mixed-mode I+II up to increment j becomes (Figure 3.5)

$$G_{\mathrm{d,m}}^j = G_{\mathrm{d,m}}^{j-1} + \sum_{i=\mathrm{I}}^{\mathrm{II}}\left(\frac{\sigma_i^{j-1}\delta_i^{j-1}}{2} + \delta G_i^j - \frac{\sigma_i^j\delta_i^j}{2}\right) \tag{3.18}$$

which leads to

$$G_{\mathrm{d,m}}^j = G_{\mathrm{d,m}}^{j-1} + \sum_{i=\mathrm{I}}^{\mathrm{II}}\left(\frac{\sigma_i^{j-1}\delta_i^j - \sigma_i^j\delta_i^{j-1}}{2}\right) \tag{3.19}$$

Equation (3.19) represents the energy dissipated in mixed-mode I+II at a given increment j calculating the mode I and II contributions. The energetic criterion based on the power law

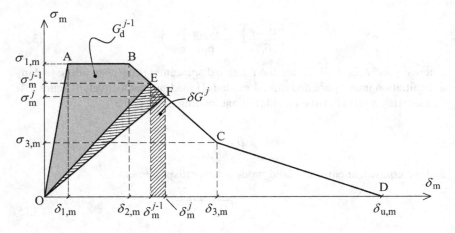

FIGURE 3.5 Evaluation of mixed-mode I+II fracture energy increment in the second softening branch of the cohesive law.

$$\left(\frac{G_{\mathrm{I}}}{G_{\mathrm{Ic}}}\right)^{\gamma} + \left(\frac{G_{\mathrm{II}}}{G_{\mathrm{IIc}}}\right)^{\gamma} = 1 \tag{3.20}$$

is employed to simulate fracture propagation under general mixed-mode I+II loading. Considering

$$\alpha = \frac{G_{\mathrm{II}}}{G_{\mathrm{I}}} \quad \text{and} \quad G_{\mathrm{T}} = G_{\mathrm{I}} + G_{\mathrm{II}} = G_{\mathrm{I}}(1+\alpha) \tag{3.21}$$

the total critical fracture energy at failure (G_{Tc}) for a given mode ratio (α) becomes

$$G_{\mathrm{Tc}} = \frac{G_{\mathrm{Ic}} G_{\mathrm{IIc}} (1+\alpha)}{\left[G_{\mathrm{IIc}}^{\gamma} + \left(\alpha G_{\mathrm{Ic}}\right)^{\gamma} \right]^{1/\gamma}} \tag{3.22}$$

Equation (3.22) can also be used to obtain the total energy (i.e., under mixed-mode I+II loading) dissipated at the inflection points B and C (Figure 3.5) from the corresponding values under pure mode loading. At point B, the components (I and II) of the dissipated fracture energy are given by

$$G_{\mathrm{d},i(\mathrm{B})} = \frac{k\delta_{1,i}\left(\delta_{2,i} - \delta_{1,i}\right)}{2} \; ; \; i = \mathrm{I}, \mathrm{II} \tag{3.23}$$

where $\delta_{1,i}$ is the relative displacement under mode i at damage onset obtained from the respective local strengths ($\sigma_{1,i}$) and $\delta_{2,i}$ is the relative displacement under mode i at the inflection point B. The total energy dissipated under mixed-mode I+II at point B (i.e., $G_{\mathrm{d,m(B)}}$) is obtained from Eq. (3.22) considering the $G_{\mathrm{d},i(\mathrm{B})}$ values ($i = \mathrm{I}, \mathrm{II}$) at point B in place of the respective G_{ic}. The corresponding mixed-mode relative displacement becomes

$$\delta_{2,\mathrm{m}} = \frac{2G_{\mathrm{d,m(B)}}}{k\delta_{1,\mathrm{m}}} + \delta_{1,\mathrm{m}} \tag{3.24}$$

Following the same procedure, the fracture energy components at point C are given by

$$G_{\mathrm{d},i(\mathrm{C})} = \frac{k\delta_{1,i}\left(\delta_{2,i} - \delta_{1,i} + \delta_{3,i}\right)}{2} - \frac{\sigma_{3,i}\delta_{2,i}}{2} \; ; \; i = \mathrm{I}, \mathrm{II} \tag{3.25}$$

The same relation can be applied considering mixed-mode I+II loading allowing to obtain the mixed-mode relative displacement at point C,

$$\delta_{3,\mathrm{m}} = \frac{2G_{\mathrm{d,m(C)}} + \sigma_{3,\mathrm{m}}\delta_{2,\mathrm{m}}}{k\delta_{1,\mathrm{m}}} - \delta_{2,\mathrm{m}} + \delta_{1,\mathrm{m}} \tag{3.26}$$

where $\sigma_{3,m}$ is defined from its stress components in mode I and II using the quadratic stress criterion (Eq. 3.12):

$$\sigma_{3m} = \frac{\sigma_{3,I}\sigma_{3,II}\sqrt{1+\beta^2}}{\sqrt{\sigma_{3,II}^2 + \beta^2\sigma_{3,I}^2}} \tag{3.27}$$

The total fracture energy in each mode G_{ic} ($i =$ I, II) is obtained from the area circumscribed by the trapezoidal-bilinear cohesive law for pure modes, which gives

$$G_{ic} = \frac{k\delta_{1,i}\left(\delta_{2,i} - \delta_{1,i} + \delta_{3,i}\right)}{2} + \frac{\sigma_{3,i}\left(\delta_{u,i} - \delta_{2,i}\right)}{2} \; ; \; i = \text{I, II} \tag{3.28}$$

This relation can also be used under mixed-mode I+II loading to determine the ultimate relative displacement under mixed-mode I+II ($\delta_{u,m}$), given by

$$\delta_{u,m} = \frac{2G_{Tc} - k\delta_{1,m}(\delta_{2,m} - \delta_{1,m} + \delta_{3,m})}{\sigma_{3,m}} + \delta_{2,m} \tag{3.29}$$

The different expressions defining the damage parameter (d) of the cohesive law can now be obtained for the three softening regions applying the following mixed-mode I+II relation derived from Eq. (3.11)

$$\sigma_m^j = (1-d)k\delta_m^j \text{ for } \delta_{1,m} \le \delta_m^j \le \delta_{u,m} \tag{3.30}$$

In the horizontal plateau (line A–B, i.e., for $\delta_{1,m} \le \delta_m^j \le \delta_{2,m}$ in Figure 3.5), Eq. (3.30) can be equated to the mixed-mode local strength ($\sigma_{1,m}$), i.e., $\sigma_m = \sigma_{1,m}$. On the other hand, the local strength can also be obtained using Eq. (3.10)

$$\sigma_{1,m} = k\delta_{1,m} \tag{3.31}$$

which allows deriving the damage parameter in the plateau region

$$d = 1 - \frac{\delta_{1,m}}{\delta_m^j} \tag{3.32}$$

In the second softening branch (between points B and C, i.e., for $\delta_{2,m} \le \delta_m^j \le \delta_{3,m}$ in Figure 3.5), the damage parameter is obtained equating the actual dissipated energy (Eq. 3.19) to the area delimitated by O-A-B-E that is given by

$$G_{d,m}^j = G_{Tc} - \frac{\sigma_{3,m}(\delta_{u,m} - \delta_m^j) + \sigma_m^j\delta_{3,m}}{2} \tag{3.33}$$

Combining Eqs. (3.30) and (3.33), the evolution of the damage parameter in this softening branch yields

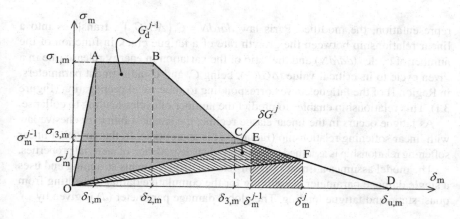

FIGURE 3.6 Evaluation of mixed-mode I+II fracture energy increment in the third softening branch of the cohesive law.

$$d = 1 + \frac{2\left(G_{d,m}^{j} - G_{Tc}\right) + \sigma_{3,m}\left(\delta_{u,m} - \delta_{m}^{j}\right)}{k\delta_{m}^{j}\delta_{3,m}} \qquad (3.34)$$

In the last softening zone (between points C and D, i.e., for $\delta_{3,m} \leq \delta_{m}^{j} \leq \delta_{u,m}$ in Figure 3.6), the area of the polygon O-A-B-C-E is equated to the actual dissipated energy (Eq. 3.19) giving rise to

$$G_{d,m}^{j} = G_{Tc} - \frac{\sigma_{m}^{j}\delta_{u,m}}{2} \qquad (3.35)$$

Substituting Eq. (3.30) in Eq. (3.35), leads to

$$d = 1 + 2\frac{G_{d,m}^{j} - G_{Tc}}{k\delta_{m}^{j}\delta_{u,m}} \qquad (3.36)$$

During softening, the damage parameter is updated incrementally during loading history, depending on the energy dissipated in the fracture process. Gradual degradation of bone material properties as function of applied loading is simulated, following the trapezoidal-bilinear cohesive law representing bone damage mechanisms in the course of its fracture process.

3.3.2.2 Fatigue/Fracture Mixed-Mode I+II CZM

A previously developed mixed-mode I+II CZM suitable to deal with high-cycle fatigue loading [de Moura et al., 2015] was applied to simulate fatigue/fracture behaviour of cortical bone tissue. The CZM is based on the modified Paris law suitable for the simulation of fatigue/fracture under different loading modes. The modified Paris law governs the steady-state damage growth occurring in the second stage of fatigue life (Region II in Figure 3.1). In a bi-logarithmic representation, the modified Paris law $da/dN = C_1\left(\Delta G/G_c\right)^{C_2}$ translates into a linear relationship between the growth rate of a fatigue crack in function of the number of cycles (da/dN) and the ratio of the variation in energy release rate in a given cycle to its critical value ($\Delta G/G_c$), being C_1 and C_2 adjustment parameters, in Region II of the fatigue curve corresponding to subcritical propagation (Figure 3.1). This relationship enables to predict the number of cycles leading to collapse.

As fatigue occurs in the linear elastic regime, the simplest bilinear cohesive law with linear softening relationship (Figure 3.7) is appropriate. In this model, a linear softening relationship is assumed to mimic gradual degradation of material properties.

The model assumes a linear traction-relative displacements softening and uses a single damage parameter accounting for the cumulative damage resulting from quasi-static and fatigue loading. The global damage parameter (d) is given by

$$d = d_s + d_f \tag{3.37}$$

being d_s and d_f the static and fatigue damage parameters, respectively, following the same softening law. The static damage parameter can be obtained equating Eq. (3.30) to the equation of the straight line defining the softening region

$$\sigma_m^j = k\delta_{I,m}^j\left(\frac{\delta_{u,m}^j - \delta_m^j}{\delta_{u,m}^j - \delta_{I,m}^j}\right) \tag{3.38}$$

which leads to

$$d_s = \frac{\delta_{u,m}^j(\delta_m^j - \delta_{I,m}^j)}{\delta_m^j(\delta_{u,m}^j - \delta_{I,m}^j)} \tag{3.39}$$

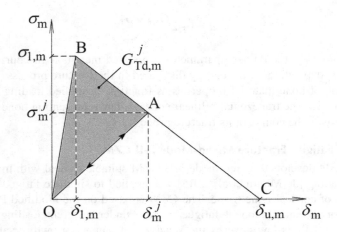

FIGURE 3.7 Cohesive law for a general mixed-mode I+II loading.

where j identifies the current increment. The fatigue damage parameter (d_f) evolves as a function of time, i.e., number of cycles (N). The rate of this evolution can be expressed as

$$\frac{d(d_f)}{dN} = \frac{d(d_f)}{d\delta^j_{m,k}} \frac{d\delta^j_{m,k}}{dA^j_{p,k}} \frac{dA^j_{p,k}}{dN} \qquad (3.40)$$

for a given integration point k. The first term of Eq. (3.40) can be obtained by differentiation of Eq. (3.39), since the same constitutive relation is adopted for static and fatigue loading

$$\frac{d(d_f)}{d\delta^j_{m,k}} = \frac{\delta^j_{u,m,k}\delta^j_{l,m,k}}{\left(\delta^j_{u,m,k}-\delta^j_{l,m,k}\right)\left(\delta^j_{m,k}\right)^2} \qquad (3.41)$$

The second term measures the evolution of the current displacement at the integration point k ($\delta^j_{m,k}$) in function of the damaged area relative to point k ($A^j_{p,k}$). This rate is obtained assuming that the ratio between $A^j_{p,k}$ and the total area ($A_{t,k}$) relative to each integration point is equal to the ratio between the dissipated energy $G^j_{Td,m,k}$ and the fracture energy for the current mode-mixity ($G^j_{Tc,k}$). From Figure 3.7, the following relation arises,

$$G^j_{Td,m,k} = G^j_{Tc,m,k} - \frac{\sigma^j_m\delta^j_{u,m,k}}{2} \qquad (3.42)$$

where

$$\sigma^j_m = \left(1-d_f\right)\frac{\sigma^j_{u,m,k}}{\delta^j_{l,m,k}}\delta^j_{m,k} \qquad (3.43)$$

taking into consideration Eq. (3.30). Combining Eqs. (3.39), (3.42) and (3.43) results [de Moura et al., 2015]

$$\frac{d\delta^j_{m,k}}{dA^j_{p,k}} = \frac{\delta^j_{u,m,k}-\delta^j_{l,m,k}}{A^j_{t,k}} \qquad (3.44)$$

The third term of Eq. (3.40) represents the local damaged area growth in function of number of cycles at the integration point k. The present high-cycle fatigue model is based on the modified Paris law, which in its general form, writes for a given increment j

$$\frac{dA^j}{dN} = C_1 \left(\frac{\Delta G^j_T}{G^j_{Tc}}\right)^{C_2} \qquad (3.45)$$

This law relates the global damage growth rate as a function of the number of cycles (dA^j/dN) with the ratio between the variation of the strain energy release rate in a cycle and the critical value for the actual mode ratio (G_{Tc}^j) with C_1 and C_2 being adjusting parameters determined experimentally. The global damage growth rate dA^j/dN can be related with the local growth rates $dA_{p,k}^j/dN$ of the several integration points (n_{CZL}) undertaking softening in the cohesive zone length,

$$\frac{dA^j}{dN} = \sum_{k=1}^{n_{CZL}} \frac{dA_{p,k}^j}{dN} \tag{3.46}$$

Applying the modified Paris law (Eq. 3.45) to local damage growth rate at a given integration point, k becomes

$$\frac{dA_{p,k}^j}{dN} = \frac{C_{1,m,k}^j r_{w,k}}{n_{CZL}} \left(\frac{\Delta G_{T,m,k}^j}{G_{Tc,m,k}^j} \right)^{C_{2,m,k}^j} \tag{3.47}$$

where $r_{w,k}$ is the relative weight of the actual integration point k in the used integration scheme [de Moura et al., 2014] and $C_{1,m,k}^j$, $C_{2,m,k}^j$ the fatigue parameters for the current mode ratio. Defining the load ratio in a cycle as $R = P_{min}/P_{max}$ and taken into account that $G=f(P^2)$ (see Eq. 3.5), it can be written

$$R^2 = \frac{G_{T,min,k}^j}{G_{T,max,k}^j} \tag{3.48}$$

The variation of total strain energy release rate in a cycle should be given by [Donough et al., 2015]

$$\Delta G_{T,k}^j = \left(\sqrt{G_{T,max,k}^j} - \sqrt{G_{T,min,k}^j} \right)^2 \tag{3.49}$$

Combining Eqs. (3.48) and (3.49) results

$$\Delta G_{T,k}^j = (1-R)^2 G_{T,max,k}^j \tag{3.50}$$

The value of maximum strain energy release rate in a given integration point k for each increment j under mixed-mode I+II loading ($G_{T,max,k}^j$) is achieved adding the mode I and mode II components. These components are continuously updated during load incrementation employing the trapezoidal rule

$$G_{i,k}^j = G_{i,k}^{j-1} + \frac{\sigma_{i,k}^{j-1} + \sigma_{i,k}^j}{2} (\delta_{i,k}^j - \delta_{i,k}^{j-1}) \; ; \; (i = \text{I, II}) \tag{3.51}$$

i.e., by making the product between the variation of the relative displacement in consecutive increments ($j-1$ and j) and the average traction in mode i (i = I,

II). Assuming the linear energetic criterion (Eq. 3.20 with $\gamma = 1$) and taking into account that

$$G_{T,k}^j = G_{I,k}^j + G_{II,k}^j = G_{I,k}^j(1+\alpha_k^j) \quad \text{being} \quad \alpha_k^j = \frac{G_{II,k}^j}{G_{I,k}^j} \tag{3.52}$$

yields,

$$G_{Tc,k}^j = \frac{G_{Ic}G_{IIc}(1+\alpha_k^j)}{G_{IIc} + \alpha_k^j G_{Ic}} \tag{3.53}$$

This equation establishes that mode-mixity can be different for the several integration points undergoing damage and can alter between consecutive increments for each integration point. Consequently, the modified Paris law constants $C_{1,m,k}^j$ and $C_{2,m,k}^j$ depend on the current mode-mixity at point k. These parameters can be related with the pure mode ones ($C_{1,I}$, $C_{1,II}$, $C_{2,I}$ and $C_{2,II}$), employing the following relations that provide the variation of the modified Paris law coefficients as a function of mode-mixity [Moreira et al., 2015]

$$\ln(C_{1,m,k}^j) = \ln(C_{1,I}) + \frac{\left[\ln(C_{1,II}) - \ln(C_{1,I})\right]G_{II,k}^j}{G_{T,k}^j}$$

$$\tag{3.54}$$

$$C_{2,m,k}^j = C_{2,I} + \frac{(C_{2,II} - C_{2,I})G_{II,k}^j}{G_{T,k}^j}$$

The evolution of the damage parameter d_f as a function of increment of number of cycles ΔN can now be obtained by replacing Eqs. (3.41), (3.44) and (3.47) into Eq. (3.40),

$$\Delta d_f(\Delta N) = \frac{\delta_{u,m,k}^j \delta_{1,m,k}^j C_{1,m,k}^j r_{w,k}}{A_{t,k} n_{CZL} \left(\delta_{m,k}^j\right)^2} \left(\frac{\Delta G_{T,k}^j}{G_{Tc,k}^j}\right)^{C_{2,m,k}^j} \Delta N \tag{3.55}$$

The cycle jump ΔN should be chosen under the compromise of results accuracy and minimisation of the computational effort, i.e., it should be defined as being the maximum value leading to convergence. In general, values around $\Delta d_{fmax} = 0.5\%$ lead to cycle jumps ΔN producing convergent solutions in acceptable CPU time consuming.

This relation is implemented in cohesive zone elements and permits the simulation of gradual material properties degradation under mixed-mode I+II loading as a function of the number of cycles in high-cycle fatigue problems. This model can be considered a valuable tool to estimate the materials fatigue life and it will be applied in the context of fatigue of cortical bone tissue in the following sections.

3.4 SUMMARY

The application of fracture mechanics concepts to cortical bone tissue is a valid strategy to study its fracture behaviour. In this context, the development of appropriate cohesive zone models for the quasi-static fracture and fatigue/fracture behaviour of cortical bone tissue is quite relevant due to the non-linear fracture behaviour of this material dictated by the development of a non-negligible fracture process zone. In this chapter, a mixed-mode I+II cohesive zone model considering trapezoidal-bilinear softening law appropriate for quasi-static fracture analysis is developed. A simpler version, i.e., a bilinear law with linear softening, is presented for fatigue analysis since fatigue occurs in the linear elastic regime.

4 Mode I Fracture Characterisation

Mode I loading is also known as the "opening mode", and it is characterised by inducing tensile loading at the crack tip. Fracture characterisation under mode I loading can be achieved by means of specific specimens where remote applied loading induces pure opening mode I at the crack tip.

The strength and the fracture toughness of cortical bone are affected by its constituents (e.g., mineral, collagen and water) and microstructural factors such as vascular porosity, size, shape, orientation and density of osteons, interstitial matrix and cement line [Yeni et al., 2000; Granke et al., 2016]. The role of these microstructural constituents in the cortical bone fracture is crucial. Indeed, organic collagen is known to play an important role in bone's permanent deformation affecting plasticity and toughness. Dry bone is more brittle [Morais et al., 2010] because dry collagen has lost its capacity for deformation and energy absorption. In addition, the cement line, which is the thin mineralised layer that surrounds the external layer of each osteon, has inferior mechanical properties when compared to osteon and matrix. This microstructural component is a 1 to 2·m-thick layer of mineralised matrix deficient in collagen fibres and plays a vital role in the microstructural heterogeneity and the fracture resistance of the cortical bone tissue. In fact, it has a greater degree of low toughness mineral contents and behaves as a brittle material. The cement lines accumulate micro-damage since they are weaker pathways to fracture, constituting favourable domains for micro-cracking nucleation in the early stage of the loading process, being generally disposed along the longitudinal axis of long bones. In effect, longitudinal fractures generally take place along the cement lines and are the easiest to occur. Thereby, the cement lines are the preferred/weaker cracking path leading to crack deflection. Consequently, the higher the proportion of interstitial bone region in the cortical bone, the higher the risk of fracture and lower the fracture resistance. Moreover, the higher density of vascular and Volkmann canals results in an accelerated growth rate of fracture and failure in cortical bone, since these canals act as stress concentrators by which crack propagation path might be deflected. These voids may decrease drastically the bone failure load-bearing capacity, since they are the main source of initiation and coalescence of micro-cracks. As a consequence of increasing load level or fatigue loading, the developed micro-cracks tend to coalesce and form macro-cracks that deflect along the cement lines and circumvent the cylindrical osteons. Thus, fracture toughness is mostly influenced at the microscope level by micro-crack trajectories within the weakest microstructural path and highly increases when the crack deflects and twists. The interaction of crack with the cement lines leads to several damaging mechanisms

DOI: 10.1201/9781003375081-4

occurring at the fracture process zone, as is the case of crack deflection and bifurcation, and osteons pull-out mimicking a "fibre-bridging" failure phenomenon. These features are beneficial as they contribute to increasing bone toughness and transforming bone fracture in a non-linear fracture mechanics problem.

In contrast to longitudinal fracture, the transverse one starts perpendicular to the cement line, but it deflects and propagates along the weaker region (i.e., cement line) after a small growth since fractures tend to take the path of least resistance. In fact, the higher the mechanical resistance of the osteon, the higher the force to fracture, or in other words, more energy is necessary for crack propagation. Hence, the fracture toughness, which represents the mechanical property that quantifies cortical bone resistance to crack initiation and propagation, is higher for crack propagation perpendicular to the osteons (transverse cross-section) as compared to crack propagation parallel to the osteons (longitudinal cross-section) [Behiri et al., 1989; Feng et al., 2000]. In the longitudinal direction, the crack propagates almost along the mode I plane, which requires lesser energy to propagate, giving rise to flatten *Resistance*-curves (*R*-curves) after some propagation. In more drastic situations, a complete transverse bone fracture can occur when the crack penetrates the osteons. In such cases, the energy required for crack propagation increases mainly due to the crack deflection mechanism, which leads to the monotonic rising trend of the *R*-curves. Yadav et al. [2021] observed that crack initiation toughness in the transverse orientation is about five times higher than in the longitudinal orientation, whereas the crack growth toughness in the transverse orientation is about 23 times higher than in the longitudinal orientation.

In consequence of the discussed statements, bone tissue fracture occurs predominantly in the TL or RL fracture system, where the first letter identifies the direction perpendicular to the crack plane and the second one the direction of crack propagation. In fact, the cortical bone planes LR and LT (Figure 4.1) are prone to suffer fractures owing to less material resistance in directions perpendicular to the osteons. In view of the almost transverse isotropic behaviour of bone discussed in Chapter 2, it is expected that the fracture toughness of those fracture systems will be similar. Considering the specificities of the cortical bone tissue (thin shell shape), it is easier to get specimens for characterisation in the TL fracture system (Figure 4.1).

Fracture characterisation of cortical bone tissue under mode I loading has been addressed by considering several different tests. Bone size, its anatomy and geometry limit the specimen dimensions. The most commonly employed are the compact tension (CT) and the single-edge-notched beam (SENB) tests, which will be discussed in more detail. The single-layer compact sandwich (Figure 4.2a) can be considered a variant of the CT test, consisting of bonding a pair of metallic plates to a thin strip of notched bone in order to increase its stiffness [Wang et al., 1998; Phelps et al., 2000]. The chevron-notched beam (Figure 4.2b) [Zioupos and Currey, 1998; Yan et al., 2006] is a variant of the SENB test and relies on the consideration of a triangular chevron ligament (triangular isosceles cross-section),

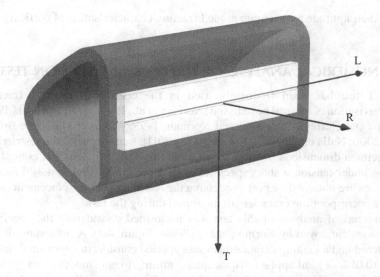

FIGURE 4.1 Specimen obtained for characterisation in the TL fracture system.

making the stored elastic energy proportional to the square of the load [Tattersall and Tappin, 1996].

The CT and SENB tests are the most commonly used tests in the context of mode I fracture characterisation. Therefore, a detailed numerical analysis considering cohesive zone modelling is presented in the following, aiming to critically

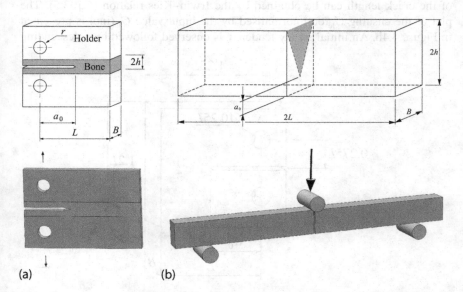

FIGURE 4.2 Schematic representations of the tests: (a) single-layer compact sandwich and (b) chevron-notched beam.

assess their aptitude for accurate mode I fracture characterisation of cortical bone tissue.

4.1 NUMERICAL ANALYSIS OF THE COMPACT TENSION TEST

The CT test has been frequently used in the context of mode I fracture characterisation of cortical bone tissue [Norman et al., 1996; Vashishth et al., 1997; Zioupos and Currey, 1998; Yeni and Norman, 1998; Akkus et al., 2000; Brown et al., 2000; Nalla et al., 2004; Koester et al., 2011], mainly due to the restrictions on specimen dimensions possible to get from this material. This test consists of loading under tension a short specimen with a pre-crack (Figure 4.3). Fracture properties are obtained by post-processing the resulting load–displacement curve and the corresponding crack length measured during the test.

A numerical analysis of this test was performed considering the specimen dimensions employed by Norman et al., [1996] (Figure 4.3). A refined mesh was considered and a loading displacement was applied considering very small increments (0.01% of total applied displacement) aiming to get smooth crack growth. Typical elastic (Table 4.1) and fracture (Table 4.2) properties [Pereira et al., 2012] of bovine cortical bone tissue were used in the simulations.

The load–displacement curve and the respective crack length are recorded in the course of the analysis aiming to obtain the compliance versus crack length relationship, $C = f(a)$. A third-degree polynomial (Figure 4.4a) was adjusted with good correlation to the function $C = f(a)$ to get the dC/da relation after differentiation. The evolution of the critical strain energy release rate as a function of the crack length can be obtained by the Irwin–Kies relation (Eq. 3.5). The plot of the ensuing $G_{Ic}(out)$ normalised by the input value $G_{Ic}(inp)$ is presented in Figure 4.4b. An initial steady tendency is observed followed by a descending

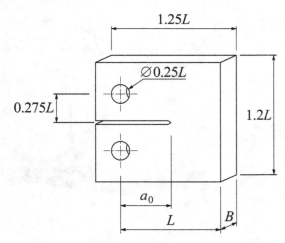

FIGURE 4.3 Schematic representation of the CT test with dimensions in mm, $L = 14$, $B = 3$, $2h = 1.2L = 16.8$ and $a_0 = 7$ [adapted from Norman et al., 1996].

TABLE 4.1

Elastic Properties Used in the Numerical Models for Bovine Bone [Pereira et al., 2012]

	E_L (MPa)	E_R (MPa)	E_T (MPa)	ν_{LR}	ν_{LT}	ν_{RT}	G_{LR} (MPa)	G_{LT} (MPa)	G_{RT} (MPa)
Cortical bone	20,880	9,550	9,550	0.37	0.37	0.37	2,150	4,740	4,740

TABLE 4.2

Cohesive Properties of Bovine Bone [Pereira et al., 2012]

	$\delta_{1,I}=\delta_{2,I}$ (mm)	$\sigma_{1,I}$ (MPa)	$\delta_{3,I}$ (mm)	$\sigma_{3,I}$ (MPa)	G_{Ic} (N/mm)
Cortical bone	3.6E−5	36.0	0.07	4.9	1.77

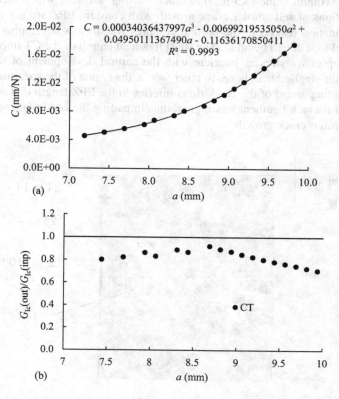

FIGURE 4.4 Results of CT test simulation: (a) $C = f(a)$ relationship adjusted by polynomial with third degree and (b) the resulting G_{Ic}(out) normalised by the input value G_{Ic}(inp).

trend after some crack growth. However, the small plateau value points to a ratio $G_{Ic}(\text{out})/G_{Ic}(\text{inp})$ of about 0.8, meaning that this test is not adequate for a truthful fracture characterisation of bone. In fact, the input value is not properly captured after post-processing the results ensuing from the numerical analysis.

A more detailed analysis of the fracture process was done aiming to explain the observed inaccuracy. Figure 4.5 shows the outline of the normal stress-inducing mode I fracture ahead of the crack tip. It can be verified that the profile of normal positive stresses ahead of the crack tip is confined in length due to the presence of compressive stresses developing beyond the neutral axis. This phenomenon is becoming aggravated with the reduction of the ligament length as consequence of crack growth and it leads to non-self-similar crack propagation.

These results can be confirmed in Figure 4.6, which plots the evolution of the cohesive zone length (CZL) as a function of the propagated crack during the test. The CZL is constituted by the set of integration points under softening in the cohesive zone law and is a simplified representation of the volumetric non-negligible fracture process zone (FPZ) that develops in quasi-brittle materials during fracture. In Figure 4.6, it can be observed that CZL diminishes monotonically, from a maximum value (3.5 mm) at crack-starting advance, which means that the conditions of self-similar crack growth with constant FPZ are not fulfilled. The explanation resides in the normal compressive stresses developing beyond the neutral axis due to bending. The short ligament length of the CT implies that those compressive stresses interfere with the natural development of the FPZ, which is non-negligible in bone. In other words, the region of the specimen under tensile loading ahead of the crack tip is inferior to the FPZ length that would be developed if crack ligament was higher, thus impeding the conditions necessary for self-similar crack growth.

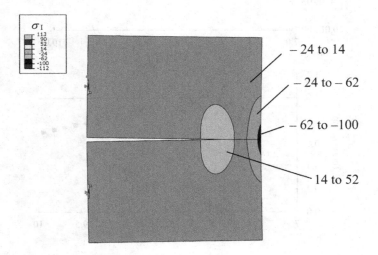

FIGURE 4.5 Profile of normal stresses (in MPa) inducing mode I facture ahead of the crack tip.

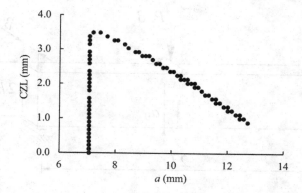

FIGURE 4.6 Evolution of the CZL as a function of crack growth in the CT test.

4.2 NUMERICAL ANALYSIS OF THE SINGLE-EDGE-NOTCHED BEAM TEST

The SENB test consists of a specimen with a vertical pre-crack at the mid-span under three-point bending (Figure 4.7). Due to applied loading, crack tends to propagate vertically under tensile loading induced by bending.

A finite element analysis was performed considering a refined mesh. Loading displacement was applied with small increments (0.01% of total applied displacement), aiming to get smooth propagation. The mechanical properties were the same as those used in the analysis of the CT test. The numerical load–displacement data and the corresponding crack lengths were duly registered during the test in order to obtain the $C = f(a)$ relationship, to which a third polynomial function was adjusted (Figure 4.8) to perform differentiation. Applying the Irwin–Kies relation (Eq. 3.5) allows us to obtain the evolution of the normalised critical strain energy release rate as a function of the crack length. It can be verified that the resulting values ($G_{Ic}(out)$) are clearly below the entered one ($G_{Ic}(inp)$), which reveals a malfunction of this fracture test.

A finer study was performed on the SENB test. Analysing the outline of the normal stresses in the vicinity of the crack tip, a phenomenon similar to the one that occurred in the CT test can be observed. Actually, the normal compressive stresses induced by bending above the neutral axis (Figure 4.9) constrain the natural development of the FPZ. This statement can be confirmed in Figure 4.10, which shows a gradual decrease of the CZL as the crack propagates, proving that the conditions of self-similar crack growth are not satisfied in the SENB test. This circumstance precludes an accurate determination of the fracture energy under mode I loading with the SENB test.

In summary, it can be concluded that because of the complex microstructure and composition of cortical bone tissue, a non-negligible FPZ due to micro-cracking, crack deviation and fibre-bridging develops ahead of the crack tip. These issues and the natural limitations associated with the size of specimens possible

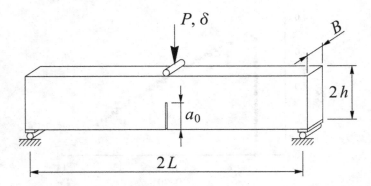

FIGURE 4.7 Geometry of the SENB specimen analyzed with dimensions (in mm): $2L = 16$, $B = 2$, $2h = 4$ and $a_0 = 2$.

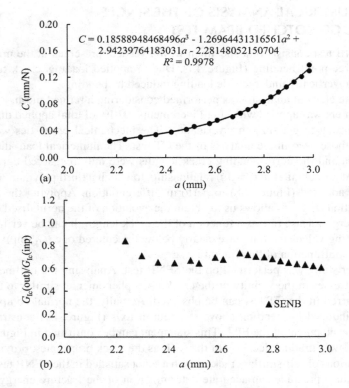

FIGURE 4.8 Results of SENB test simulation: (a) $C = f(a)$ relationship adjusted by polynomial with third degree and (b) the resulting $G_{Ic}(\text{out})$ normalised by the input value $G_{Ic}(\text{inp})$.

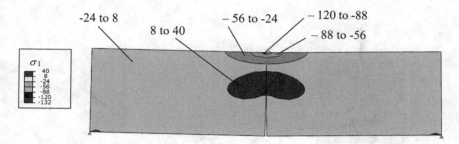

FIGURE 4.9 Profile of normal stresses (in MPa) inducing mode I facture ahead of the crack tip.

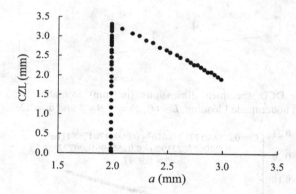

FIGURE 4.10 Evolution of the CZL as a function of crack length in the SENB test.

to get in bone render difficulty in the definition of tests appropriate for accurate bone fracture characterisation.

4.3 NUMERICAL ANALYSIS OF THE DOUBLE CANTILEVER BEAM (DCB) TEST

In light of the drawbacks revealed by CT and SENB tests on the accurate estimation of the cortical bone fracture properties under mode I loading, a similar numerical analysis is performed in this section on a miniaturised version of the DCB test. The nominal specimen dimensions for bone fracture characterisation of the TL fracture system are presented in Figure 4.11.

The DCB test can be considered similar to the CT one, being the difference in the ratio length/thickness of the specimen that is quite greater in DCB, thus being considered as a "beam"-type specimen. The numerical analysis followed the same procedure described for the two previous tests. The $C = f(a)$ relation was adjusted by means of a third-degree polynomial (Figure 4.12a) to apply the Irwin–Kies formula (Eq. 3.5) and obtain the critical strain energy release rate as a function of crack length (Figure 4.12b). In this case, a stable plateau is obtained

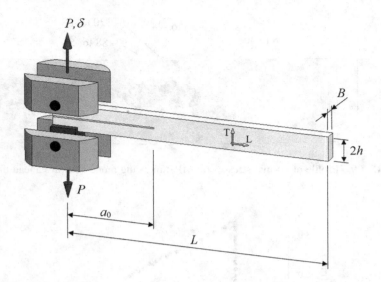

FIGURE 4.11 DCB specimen dimensions (in mm) available for bone fracture characterisation under mode I loading: $L = 60$, $2h = 6$, $B = 3$ and $a_0 = 22$.

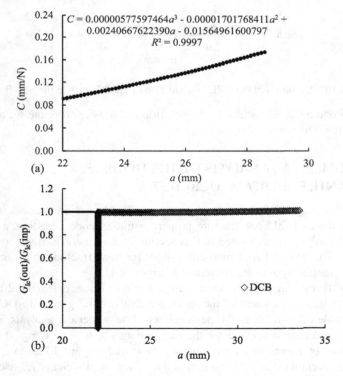

FIGURE 4.12 Results of DCB test simulation: (a) $C = f(a)$ relationship adjusted by polynomial with third degree and (b) the resulting G_{Ic}(out) normalised by the input value G_{Ic}(inp).

during crack growth with the resulting value G_{Ic}(out) in close agreement with the value considered as input, G_{Ic}(inp).

For the purpose of explaining this good result, the profile of the normal stress-inducing mode I loading at the crack tip was analysed at two different stages of crack propagation (Figure 4.13). Similar outlines can be observed, owing to the absence of any restriction to the free development of the FPZ. In fact, the long ligament length provides the necessary self-similar crack growth conditions with almost constant CZL ahead of the crack tip (Figure 4.14). This result reflects an ideal circumstance for truthful fracture characterisation of bone making the DCB test the most suitable in this context. In fact, the DCB specimen propitiates a longer length for self-similar crack propagation without undertaking spurious effects.

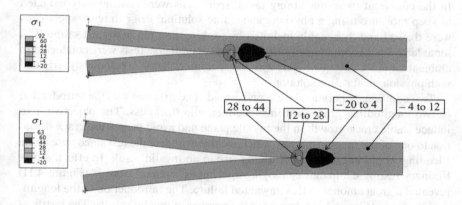

FIGURE 4.13 Profile of normal stresses (in MPa) inducing mode I facture ahead of the crack tip at two different stages of crack propagation.

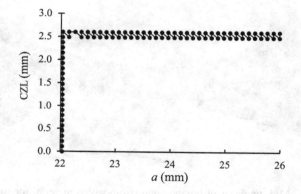

FIGURE 4.14 Evolution of the CZL as a function of crack length in the DCB test.

4.4   DCB FRACTURE TESTS

Cortical bone from the bovine femora of young animals was used for the DCB test campaign. The material was acquired from a local slaughterhouse, within a one-day post-mortem period. The sex of the animals was not known and the ages were about eight months. A longitudinal–transverse section was dissected from the interior medial region of the mid-diaphysis of each femur (Figure 4.15) and immediately cleaned, removing all the attached muscles and marrow. All the referred operations were performed with specimens being irrigated with a physiological saline solution. Subsequently, these small parts were wrapped in gauze saturated in physiological saline solution and frozen at −20°C. Before the subsequent machining operations, the piece has been unfrozen at room temperature for a period of not less than two hours. The next milling and cutting operations gave rise to the specimen nominal dimensions (L, B, $2h$) presented in Figure 4.16. In the course of these machining tasks, specimens were continuously irrigated to keep moisture using a physiological saline solution. Prior to tests, specimens were thawed and thoroughly hydrated by soaking in a physiological saline (PS) for at least 5 h at room temperature in airtight containers. Tests were conducted in ambient air (25°C, 20–40% RH) with the specimens being continuously irrigated with physiological saline solution.

Two additional operations were performed. The first one was the introduction of two longitudinal grooves at the specimen mid-thickness. The objective is to induce stable crack growth in the middle plane and avoid premature crack deviation to one of the specimen arms, which would invalidate the test since pure mode I loading would not be assured, giving rise to an invalid result. In effect, a preliminary testing campaign employing specimens without grooves (Figure 4.11) revealed a great amount of this unwanted failure. The introduction of the longitudinal grooves (Figure 4.16) decreases the number of invalid results. The justification relies on the local reduction of the resistant section width that induces easier crack propagation at the intended plane, maintaining nearly the total stiffness of

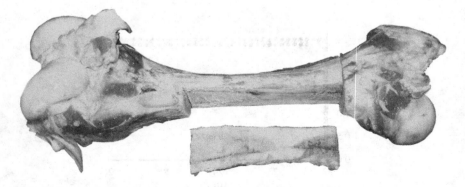

FIGURE 4.15   Mid-diaphysis of bovine femur from which material for specimens was extracted.

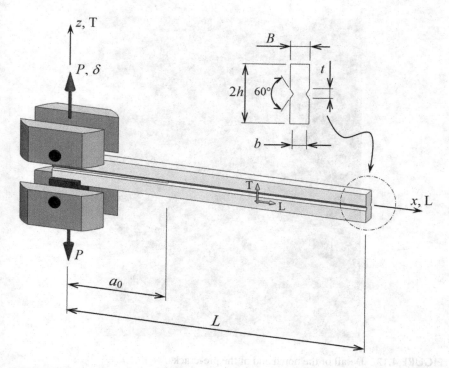

FIGURE 4.16 Schematic representation of the DCB specimen (dimensions in mm) used for mode I fracture characterisation of bone: $L = 60$, $2h = 6$, $B = 3$, $b = 2$, $t = 1$, $a_0 = 22$.

the specimen members. The final operation consisted of the introduction of the pre-crack a_0 (Figure 4.16) that followed two main steps. First, a notch (0.3 mm thickness) was machined using a circular diamond saw. Then, the pre-crack was created by means of a sharp razor blade mounted in a servo-electrical testing machine (Micro-Tester INSTRON 5848). This was accomplished by moving the actuator 0.25 mm towards the root of the notch with a velocity of 100 mm/s. This process usually reproduces natural cracks in a realistic way. This is an important aspect since blunt pre-cracks induce an unrealistic increase of fracture energy at the crack-starting advance [Morais et al., 2010]. Figure 4.17 presents an example of the created notch and pre-crack.

The experimental DCB tests (Figure 4.18) were performed using the Micro-Tester INSTRON 5848 servo-electrical testing system under displacement control imposing an actuator velocity of 0.2 mm/min, aiming to induce smooth crack propagation. The opening loading displacement (Figure 4.18) was applied to the specimen through two steel cylindrical pin-hole connections inducing mode I loading at the crack tip. The tests were performed under typical environmental laboratorial conditions, i.e., 65% relative humidity at 20°C. Load–displacement (P–δ) curves were registered with an acquisition rate of 5 Hz (Figure 4.19).

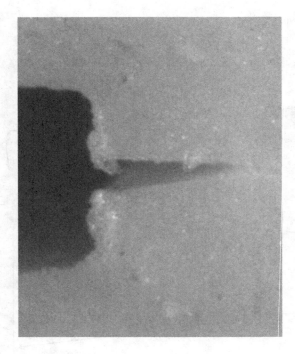

FIGURE 4.17 Detail of the notch and of the pre-crack.

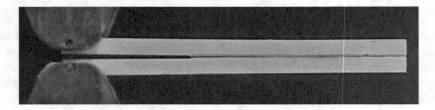

FIGURE 4.18 A photograph showing a DCB test in cortical bone tissue.

A post-processing analysis of data ensuing from the load–displacement curves is required to assess the bone fracture energy under mode I loading. Classical data reduction schemes (e.g., compliance calibration method – ISO 15024:2001) also require crack length monitoring during the test. However, the existence of a non-negligible fracture process zone with several damaging mechanisms already discussed makes impractical an accurate recording of the crack length in the course of the test (Figure 4.20). In this context, an alternative data reduction scheme based on beam theory, specimen compliance and crack equivalent concept has been employed.

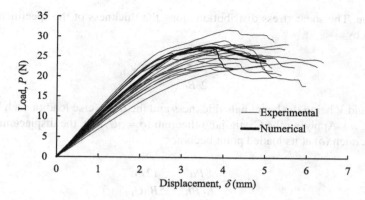

FIGURE 4.19 Load–displacement curves of the quasi-static DCB tests.

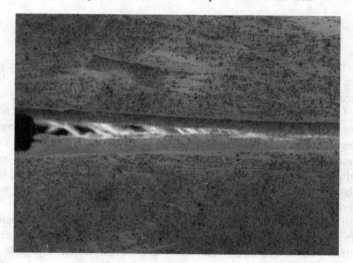

FIGURE 4.20 Detail of the crack, highlighting the pronounced fibre-bridging and consequent difficulties in identification of crack length during propagation.

4.4.1 COMPLIANCE-BASED BEAM METHOD (CBBM) APPLIED TO DCB

The method considers the Timoshenko beam theory to establish the relationship between the specimen compliance $C = \delta/P$ and current crack length, a. Assuming that specimen arms are two cantilever beams clamped at the crack tip, the strain energy due to bending and shear effects can be written as [Morais et al., 2010]

$$U = 2\left[\int_0^a \frac{M_f^2}{2E_L I}dx + \int_0^a \int_{-h/2}^{h/2} \frac{\tau^2}{2G_{LT}}B\,dy\,dx\right] \quad (4.1)$$

where M_f is the bending moment, I is the second moment of the cross-section area, E_L is the longitudinal elastic modulus and G_{LT} is the shear modulus in the

LT plane. The shear stress distribution along the thickness of the specimen arm is given by

$$\tau = \frac{3}{2} \frac{V}{Bh}\left(1 - \frac{y^2}{c^2}\right)$$ (4.2)

with c and V being the beam half-thickness and the transverse load in each beam ($0 \le x \le a$). Applying the Castigliano theorem ($\delta = \partial U / \partial P$), the displacement of the specimen (δ) at its loaded point becomes

$$\delta = \frac{8Pa^3}{E_{\mathrm{L}}Bh^3} + \frac{12Pa}{5BhG_{\mathrm{LT}}}$$ (4.3)

which leads to

$$C = \frac{8a^3}{E_{\mathrm{L}}Bh^3} + \frac{12a}{5BhG_{\mathrm{LT}}}$$ (4.4)

Bone is a natural material with remarkable scatter in its properties. Consequently, the elastic properties vary markedly from specimen to specimen. The relevance of the second term of Eq. (4.4) is minor and a typical value of G_{LT} (Table 4.1) can be used. On the contrary, the influence of E_{L} is quite relevant and an accurate estimation of each specimen value is required. With this aim, an inverse method combining experimental data and numerical analysis can be followed. The real specimen dimensions (B and h) and the initial value of crack length (a_0) are used as input in a finite element analysis simulating the DCB test. The value of E_{L} is iteratively adjusted until the initial numerical compliance (C_0) agrees with the experimental one.

After the estimation of E_{L} by this procedure, Eq. (4.4) can be used to determine an equivalent crack length (a_e) as a function of the current compliance during the fracture test. Following this procedure, the existence of a non-negligible FPZ is indirectly taken into account, since its presence ahead of the crack tip influences the specimen compliance that is used to get the equivalent crack length. Equation (4.4) can be rewritten in the form

$$\alpha\, a_e^3 + \beta\, a_e + \gamma = 0$$ (4.5)

with the coefficients,

$$\alpha = \frac{8}{Bh^3 E_{\mathrm{L}}}\ ;\quad \beta = \frac{12}{5BhG_{\mathrm{LT}}}\ ;\quad \gamma = -C$$ (4.6)

Using the Matlab® software, the solution of the resulting cubic Eq. (4.5) is found

$$a_e = \frac{1}{6\alpha}A - \frac{2\beta}{A}$$ (4.7)

with

$$A = \left[\left(-108\gamma + 12\sqrt{3 \left(\frac{4\beta^3 + 27\gamma^2\alpha}{\alpha} \right)} \right) \alpha^2 \right]^{\frac{1}{3}} \tag{4.8}$$

Taking into consideration the width reduction at the resistant section, the Irwin–Kies equation becomes

$$G_I = \frac{P^2}{2b} \frac{dC}{da} \tag{4.9}$$

where b is the width of the mid-section resulting from the introduction of the longitudinal grooves. The combination of Eqs. (4.4) and (4.9) leads to

$$G_I = \frac{6P^2}{Bbh} \left(\frac{2a_e^2}{E_L h^2} + \frac{1}{5G_{LT}} \right) \tag{4.10}$$

The described procedure has two important advantages when compared with classical approaches employed in the context of fracture characterisation of materials. In effect, the crack length monitoring in the course of the fracture test becomes unnecessary, which is a relevant benefit owing to the difficulties inherent in doing it with the required accuracy. Second, the elastic properties' variability among different specimens is accounted for in the fracture energy determination. In addition, the presented methodology also enables to obtain a complete R-curve, which represents well the fracture process.

The described data reduction scheme based on the equivalent crack length concept was applied to the experimental DCB tests whose results are plotted in Figure 4.19. The ensuing R-curves (Figure 4.21), representative of the evolution of the strain energy release rate in function of the equivalent crack length (a_e), are obtained employing data given exclusively by the load–displacement curve.

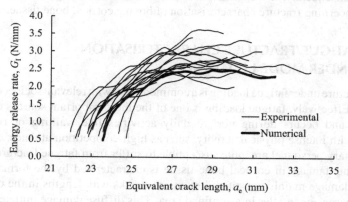

FIGURE 4.21 R-curves under mode I loading of bovine cortical bone tissue.

Apart from some undulations motivated by internal heterogeneity of cortical bone tissue affecting the fracture energy during propagation, it can be settled that two main regions are clearly identified in these curves. An initial rising trend is visible reflecting the FPZ development ahead of the pre-crack tip. When the FPZ attains its critical value, crack-starting advance takes place under self-similar conditions. This statement is reflected in the plateau trend that follows the initial rising part. In fact, steady-state crack growth with constant FPZ ahead of the crack tip for a given crack extension is a crucial condition to assure an adequate material fracture characterisation. The value given by the plateau region is representative of the fracture energy of the material under pure mode I loading, i.e., G_{Ic} values of this set of specimens of bovine cortical bone tissue are in the range of 2.0–3.0 N/mm, approximately.

In order to confirm that the proposed procedure is working properly on the determination of the fracture energies, a two-dimensional plane stress numerical analysis of the DCB test was performed considering nominal specimen dimensions (Figure 4.16), elastic properties listed in Table 4.1 and cohesive parameters representative of the fracture properties presented in Table 4.2. The exceptions were the longitudinal elastic modulus (E_L) that was determined for each specimen by the inverse procedure above described, and the fracture energy that was assumed to be the average value determined in this set of DCB samples (G_{Ic} = 2.5 N/mm) in Figure 4.21. The mesh used in the DCB simulations consists of 1908 eight-node solid plane stress elements owing to the small width B and 212 six-node cohesive elements with null thickness and a smaller width b to account for the presence of grooves. Cohesive elements were located at the specimens' mid-plane aiming to simulate damage propagation considering the quasi-static cohesive damage model described in Section 3.3.2.1. Loading displacement with small increments (0.1% of the total displacement) was applied to the specimen arms to induce stable crack growth. The numerical load–displacement curve and R-curve were included in Figures 4.19 and 4.21, respectively. It can be verified that these numerical curves reflect well the obtained experimental trends in both cases. Consequently, it was concluded that all the methodologies described are valid concerning fracture characterisation of bovine cortical bone tissue.

4.5   FATIGUE/FRACTURE CHARACTERISATION UNDER MODE I LOADING

Bone fracture under fatigue loading is a common event with relevant socioeconomic impact. Effectively, fatigue loading is one of the most important sources of bone fracture and occurs during normal daily activities like walking or running. People with intense physical activity, such as high-competition athletes, dancers and military personnel are quite susceptible to suffer from fatigue fractures.

Fatigue damage in cortical bone tissue is characterised by the formation of diffuse damage mainly constituted by micro-cracks with lengths in the order of a few microns or smaller in a confined area. This diffuse damage initiates at the sub-microscale structure (mineralised collagen fibril) and serves as a precursor for other micro-scale and larger fracture mechanisms, such as crack bridging once stable crack growth starts [Vashishth, 2007].

There are several challenges to characterise the fatigue behaviour of hard tissues, many of which are attributed to size constraints and to the complexity of their microstructure. Owing to the successful application of the DCB test in the context of quasi-static fracture characterisation of cortical bone tissue, it was decided to employ it for fatigue/fracture characterisation under pure mode I loading. The objective of the proposed methodologies is to contribute to a better understanding of the fatigue/fracture behaviour of bone and help choosing the best clinical treatment to recover or minimise the bone quality loss that is frequently the cause of painful fractures.

The experimental procedures were the same employed for quasi-static fracture characterisation. Each DCB fatigue test was performed under load control at a frequency of 2 Hz with a maximum load (P_{max}) equal to 50% of the static ultimate load (P_u). Taken into consideration that bone is a natural heterogeneous material with inherent variability, quasi-static test of each specimen prior to the fatigue test is recommended. The objective is to have a sound estimate of the static ultimate load and the fracture energy under mode I loading (G_{Ic}) by inducing a quite small crack growth. A very low displacement rate (0.075 mm/min) was applied in this quasi-static test to induce a very small crack growth nearby the maximum load (P_u). Figure 4.22 shows an example in which numerical analysis using cohesive zone models (CZM) was also included to confirm the coherence of the approach.

These quantities interfere markedly with the obtained fatigue life and they can vary significantly from specimen to specimen. Following this strategy, the effect of material scatter properties on the measured parameters diminishes. Subsequently, a fatigue test is performed in the same specimen considering the maximum load (P_{max}) equal to half of its own P_u. The load ratio in a cycle ($R = P_{min} / P_{max}$) was assumed equal to 0.1 to avoid the contact of the DCB specimen arms at unloading. During testing, the specimens were continuously irrigated to preserve hydration and prevent premature failure induced by material embrittlement (Figure 4.23). The maximum and minimum displacements in each cycle were measured aiming to calculate the evolution of the specimen compliance C

$$C = \frac{\Delta\delta}{\Delta P} = \frac{\delta_{max} - \delta_{min}}{P_{max} - P_{min}} \quad (4.11)$$

as a function of the number of cycles (N) for post-processing analysis. Several tests were performed and the large majority of them revealed stable crack growth along the specimen mid-plane (Figure 4.23).

The CBBM described in Section 4.4.1 was used to obtain the evolution of the equivalent crack length as a function of the increasing compliance and the respective strain energy release rate under mode I loading. These quantities are crucial for the definition of the modified Paris law that writes

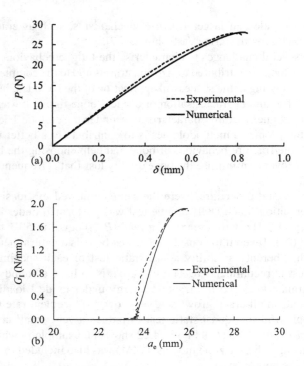

FIGURE 4.22 Experimental and numerical curves of a preliminary quasi-static DCB test on bovine cortical bone: (a) load–displacement and (b) R-curves.

$$\frac{dA_e}{dN} = C_{1,I}\left(\frac{\Delta G_I}{G_{Ic}}\right)^{C_{2,I}} = C_{1,I}\left[\frac{G_{I,max}\left(1-R\right)^2}{G_{Ic}}\right]^{C_{2,I}} \tag{4.12}$$

where $A_e = Ba_e$ is the equivalent damaged area, N is the number of cycles, R is the load ratio, in a cycle, ΔG_I and $G_{I,max}$ are the variation and maximum values of the mode I strain energy release rate in a cycle, respectively, G_{Ic} is the mode I fracture energy and $C_{1,I}$, $C_{2,I}$ are the Paris law coefficients for mode I loading.

Figure 4.24 shows an example of the main results obtained for each specimen. Figure 4.24a and 4.24b present the evolution of compliance (C) and equivalent crack length (a_e) as a function of the number of cycles (N), respectively. In both cases, a slight rising trend can be observed up to 60,000 cycles representing the gradual accumulation of damage, after which an increase of growth rate occurs leading to final failure. Similar behaviour can be observed in Figure 4.24c for the evolution of the variation of the strain energy release rate in a cycle (ΔG_I) with the number of cycles (N). Figure 4.24d plots in a bi-logarithmic scale the damaged area growth rate (dA_e/dN – mm²/cycle) as a function of the energy ratio ($\Delta G_I/G_{Ic}$) for the region of stable crack growth to which the Paris law is applicable (Figure 3.1). Although some dispersion is noticeable, there is an upward trend.

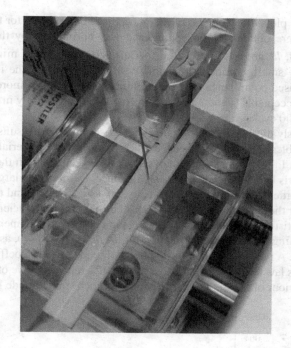

FIGURE 4.23 DCB specimen showing a crack propagating in the middle plane of the specimen during a fatigue test with continuous hydration.

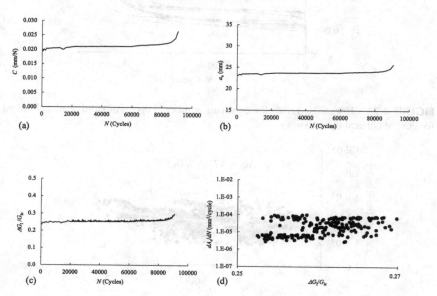

FIGURE 4.24 Evolution of (a) specimen compliance; (b) equivalent crack length; (c) variation of normalised strain energy release rate under mode I loading as a function of number of cycles; (d) damaged area growth rate as a function of energy ratio.

Figure 4.25 plots the evolution of the normalised compliance for the six valid results that were obtained. The compliance was normalised by the specimen dimensions (B, h^3 and a_0^3) according to Eq. (4.4), in order to minimise scatter induced by small variations of them. With this procedure the initial specimens' normalised compliance for $N = 0$ (Figure 4.25) becomes more consistent, revealing an acceptable scatter. The specimens failed consistently in the range of 80,000–100,000 cycles.

As previously discussed, important scatter exists in fatigue results. In cortical bone, this problem becomes aggravated since it is a natural material with inherent variability. In this context, the analysis of each specimen with the purpose of getting the Paris law coefficients lacks significance, owing to the large dispersion observed. In order to minimise this difficulty, it was decided to find the Paris law coefficients for the ensemble of all valid tests, thus obtaining coefficients more representative statistically. In this context, the results of the six specimens were postprocessed aiming to get a general relation for $dA_e/dN = f(\Delta G_I/G_{Ic})$, as can be seen in Figure 4.26. A power law was adjusted in order to identify the coefficients of the modified Paris law ($C_1 = 4.72$ mm^2/cycle, $C_2 = 8.12$), representative of the fatigue/fracture behaviour of this set of bovine bone specimens under mode I loading.

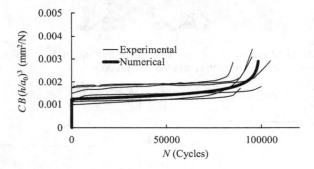

FIGURE 4.25   Normalised compliance versus number of cycles of valid results obtained for bovine cortical bone tissue.

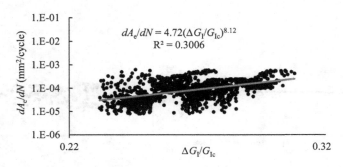

FIGURE 4.26   Bi-logarithmic representation of fatigue damage growth rate (dA_e/dN) versus $\Delta G_I/G_{Ic}$ for a set of bovine bone specimens.

TABLE 4.3

Summary of Specimen Dimensions, Young Modulus, Maximum Load, Fracture Energy and Fatigue Life for Cortical Bovine Bone Tissue

Specimen	B (mm)	$2h$ (mm)	a_0 (mm)	E_L (MPa)	P_{max} (N)	G_{Ic} (N/mm)	Fatigue life (Cycles)
1	3.8	6.5	20.5	13,720	14.0	2.0	85,326
2	4.0	6.1	21.0	14,130	11.0	1.9	96,630
3	3.6	6.7	20.5	12,600	12.0	2.6	96,645
4	3.8	6.2	22.3	13,000	10.0	1.7	81,804
5	3.7	6.4	21.0	13,500	15.0	1.8	88,740
6	3.9	6.1	20.4	12,500	15.0	2.2	87,222
Avg.	3.8	6.3	21.0	13,242	12.8	2.0	89,395
CoV (%)	3.7	3.8	3.4	4.9	16.7	16.1	6.8

Note: The smaller width b is obtained by subtracting 1 mm from B (Figure 4.16).

A finite element analysis was performed employing the cohesive zone model appropriate for fatigue loading described in Section 4.3. All the conditions considered in the quasi-static case described above (mesh, type of elements, elastic and cohesive properties, and boundary conditions) were kept. Table 4.3 lists the specimen dimensions, longitudinal Young modulus, maximum load, fracture energy and the respective fatigue lives obtained. The obtained Paris law coefficients ($C_1 = 4.72$ mm²/cycle, $C_2 = 8.12$) were considered in the cohesive zone model for high-cycle fatigue along with the average values of the geometrical and material parameters listed in Table 4.3.

The curve showing the numerical normalised compliance versus the number of cycles was obtained and included in Figure 4.25. It can be verified that the numerical curve represents well the global experimental trend, which reveals the good performance of the numerical model and the suitability of the proposed post-processing analysis of fatigue results.

4.6 SUMMARY

This chapter describes experimental and numerical works on mode I fracture of cortical bone tissue. Preliminary numerical analyses of the most common types of fracture tests led to the conclusion that the double cantilever beam is the most suitable test due to the material's fracture characteristics. Quasi-static and fatigue–fracture double cantilever beam tests were performed on hydrated cortical bone. A suitable data reduction scheme based on the equivalent crack length concept was considered to assess the evolution of the strain energy release rate during the tests. The main objectives were to determine the fracture energy under mode I loading and the fatigue life of this material. The cohesive zone models presented in Chapter 3 were used in numerical analyses in order to validate the followed experimental procedure.

5 Mode II Fracture Characterisation

Shear loading normal to the leading edge of a crack is responsible for mode II fractures. Pure shear loading can occur because of twisting or torsion efforts during normal activities [Turner et al., 2001]. A common example is the case of sudden twisting movements during sports activities that lead to frequent fractures under an almost pure shear loading. Additionally, cortical bone is weak in shear, i.e., it reveals low shear strength particularly in the longitudinal plane (longitudinal shear loading), which makes mode II fracture studies quite pertinent. Effectively, shear cracks can propagate nearly parallel to the longitudinal direction, giving rise to cleavage surfaces. In this plane, several interfaces exist at different levels, such as the interface between collagen and mineral crystals, the interface between plies or lamellae and the interface between osteons and the interstitial matrix. These interfacial regions are susceptible to delamination under shear loading, i.e., they are prone to separation of two adjacent layers or plies [Cowin, 2001], owing to the mismatch of mechanical properties of these plies. Several microstructural aspects can influence fracture under mode II loading in bone. Yeni et al. [1997] analysed the influence of porosity and osteons morphology on the mode I and mode II fracture toughness of human cortical bone. These authors concluded that porosity reduces significantly bone fracture toughness under both loading modes. In contrast, the increase of osteon density leads to a toughness increase, being more beneficial to a large number of small osteons when compared to a small number of large osteons. Tang et al. [2015] evaluated shear properties of human cortical bone at four different shear angles (0°, 30°, 60° and 90°) with respect to the long axis of the femoral shaft. They employed Iosipescu shear tests considering V-notch specimens in combination with digital image correlation for in-plane strain analysis, and fluorescence staining and laser scanning confocal microscopy for micro-crack imaging. The analysis was focused on damage mechanisms, namely on micro-cracking processes and their relationship with bone's hierarchical structures, especially the collagen fibril orientation. Similar to what happens in artificial fibre composites, inter-fibril shear damage or cracks may occur in bone during the inelastic deformation stage. In the case of 0° specimens, i.e., when shear is applied perpendicular to the bone's long axis, mineralized collagen fibrils bridge the inter-fibrous cracks making difficult their development into a major fracture. This damage mechanism leads to higher strength and strain failure when compared with other specimen orientations. For the remaining orientations (30°, 60° and 90°), it was observed that the fracture patterns are roughly aligned with the bone's long axis for all specimens. This suggests a strong structural effect on the deformation process, i.e., the shear-induced

84

DOI: 10.1201/9781003375081-5

micro-cracking of human cortical bone follows a unique pattern that is governed by the lamellar structure of the osteons.

As a consequence of these statements, fracture characterisation of cortical bone tissue under mode II loading becomes a relevant research topic. As a result of the complex fracture mechanisms described above, it becomes obvious that linear elastic fracture mechanics concepts are not appropriate to deal with mode II fracture of cortical bone tissue as occurred in the mode I case. Once again, the non-linear fracture mechanics theory via the cohesive zone model is more suitable in this context.

Fracture characterisation under mode II loading requires appropriate arrangements enabling a pure state of shear loading at the crack tip induced by the applied remote loading, which is not easy to implement. The majority of the studies are focused on the determination of the shear modulus and shear strength using the Iosipescu or Arcan tests, as it was discussed in Section 2.4. Few tests have been proposed for truthful fracture characterisation of cortical bone under pure mode II loading. Norman et al. [1996] proposed the compact shear (CS) test, which consists of a specimen similar to the one used in the CT test loading in pure shear. One of the specimen arms is fixed and the other one is loaded in the direction of the pre-crack, aiming to induce pure shear at the crack tip. Zimmerman et al. [2009, 2010] suggested the employment of the asymmetric four-point bending (AFPB) test using single-edge-notched specimens developed for general mixed-mode I+II fracture characterisation, in the context of pure mode II fracture characterisation of bone. In the following sections, these two tests and two new suggestions are subjected to detailed numerical analyses considering cohesive zone modelling. The elastic properties of bovine cortical bone (Table 4.1) were used and a typical value of $G_{IIc} = 2.0$ N/mm was considered in the numerical analysis. The goal is to evaluate their ability as valid procedures regarding mode II fracture characterisation of cortical bone tissue.

5.1   NUMERICAL ANALYSIS OF THE COMPACT SHEAR TEST

The compact shear (CS) test (Figure 5.1) is the most used for mode II fracture characterisation of cortical bone tissue [Norman et al., 1995; Norman et al., 1996; Brown et al., 2000]. Specimen dimensions are related to a given dimension H (typically 15–16 mm) as shown in Figure 5.1a). In the longitudinal direction, one of the parts of the specimen is restricted and loading displacement is applied to the other one, aiming to induce pure shear stress state at the crack tip (Figure 5.1b).

The finite element mesh used is shown in Figure 5.2. The considered dimensions, loading and boundary conditions replicate the test performed by Norman et al., [1996]. During the numerical analysis, it was verified that softening takes place near the crack tip in the cohesive elements close to the applied load (point A in Figure 5.2). This is an unwanted effect since energy is not being dissipated solely at the initial crack as it should be for an adequate fracture characterisation.

During experimental tests Norman et al., [1996] have observed unstable propagation, i.e., once crack advance begins, uncontrollable crack growth immediately

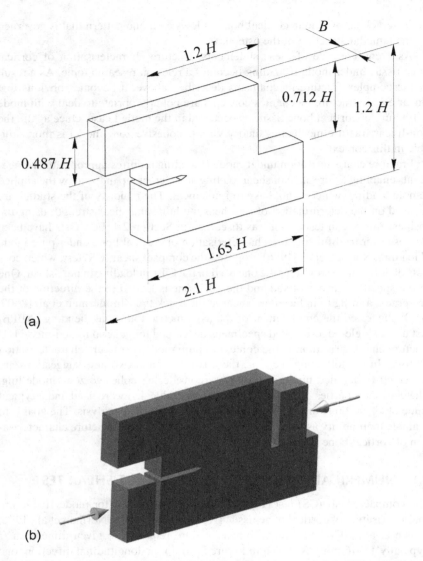

FIGURE 5.1 (a) Schematic representation of the CS specimen and (b) loading conditions.

follows causing the specimen to rupture into two parts instantaneously. This behaviour was also observed in the numerical simulations and it hindered compliance calibration as a function of crack length evolution. Instead, the compliance calibration was performed considering several virtual specimens with different initial crack lengths. A cubic polynomial was fitted to the curve $C = f(a)$ with good correlation (Figure 5.3). The found relationship was subsequently used to get an equivalent crack length during the test ($a_e = f(C)$), solving the adjusted cubic polynomial in order to a using the Matlab® software.

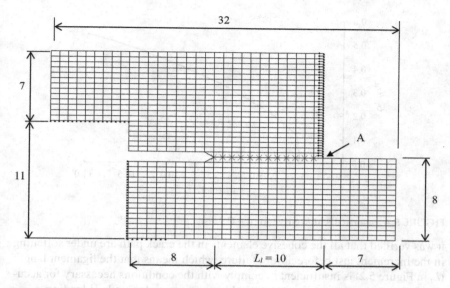

FIGURE 5.2 Mesh used in the finite element analysis for the CS test: dimensions in mm.

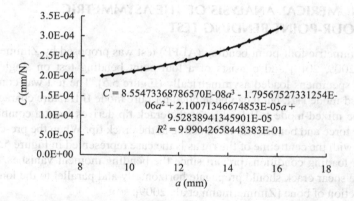

$$C = 8.55473368786570E\text{-}08a^3 - 1.79567527331254E\text{-}06a^2 + 2.10071346674853E\text{-}05a + 9.52838941345901E\text{-}05$$
$$R^2 = 9.99042658448383E\text{-}01$$

FIGURE 5.3 Compliance calibration as a function of the crack length for the CS test.

The evolution of the strain energy release rate under mode II loading as a function of a_e is calculated by means of the Irwin–Kies equation (Eq. 3.5) and is plotted in Figure 5.4. The strain energy release rate G_{II} was normalised by its critical value (G_{IIc}) in order to provide a better assessment of the difference between the obtained quantity and the one used as input in the numerical model. The normalised R-curve increases monotonically until the final failure that occurs for a G_{II}/G_{IIc} ratio inferior to unity, meaning that the value of fracture energy (G_{IIc}) used as input is not duly captured. As observed in previous mode I tests (SENB and CT), self-similar crack growth conditions are not fulfilled in the CS test. Actually,

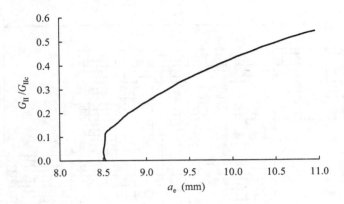

FIGURE 5.4 Normalised R-curve for the CS test.

it was verified that all the cohesive elements in the crack path are under softening in the increment just before abrupt failure, which means that the ligament length (L_l in Figure 5.2) is insufficient to comply with the conditions necessary for accurate fracture characterisation of cortical bone tissue under mode II loading.

5.2   NUMERICAL ANALYSIS OF THE ASYMMETRIC FOUR-POINT BENDING TEST

The asymmetric four-point bending (AFPB) test was proposed by Zimmermann et al., [2009, 2010] and consists of a four-point bending test on single-edge-notched specimens loaded asymmetrically (Figure 5.5). The test was conceived for mixed-mode I+II, but it can be applied for pure mode II fracture characterisation. The mixed-mode I+II loading at the crack tip derives from a combination of shear force and bending moment acting at the crack tip. When the pre-crack is aligned with the centreline of the rig as is the case represented in Figure 5.5, pure mode II loading conditions prevail since the bending moment vanishes. In this case, the shear crack should propagate horizontally and parallel to the longitudinal direction of bone [Zimmermann et al., 2009].

A finite element analysis was performed for the case of pure mode II loading (Figure 5.5 and Figure 5.6). The three upper cylinders are connected by a "rigid beam-type restriction" and a loading displacement is applied to the central one. Cohesive zone elements were inserted at the specimen mid-plane to simulate the damage growth under mode II loading conditions. Figure 5.6 shows the numerically observed failure for the conditions specified for mode II fracture characterisation.

An analysis of stress component profiles was performed at two stages: just before damage onset and just before clear crack growth (Figure 5.7), both on the longitudinal (horizontal) directions. Two important remarks can be made. First, the presence of mode I stress component (σ_I) at the crack tip is similar to the mode II component (σ_{II}) just before damage onset (Figure 5.7a), meaning that

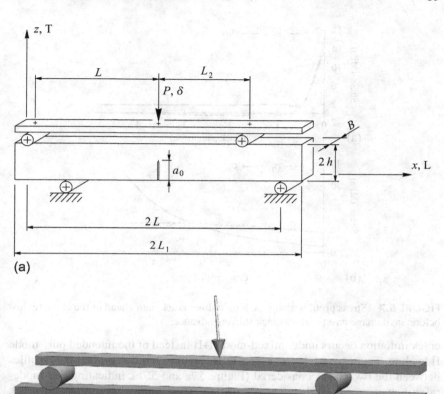

(a)

(b)

FIGURE 5.5 (a) Schematic representation of the AFPB test with, $2L_1 = 72.0$, $2L = 68.0$, $L_2 = 24.0$, $2h = 4.0$, $a_0 = h$, $B = 2.5$ (all in mm) and (b) loading conditions.

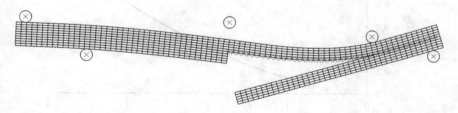

FIGURE 5.6 Numerical simulation of the AFPB test under mode II loading, showing crack propagation.

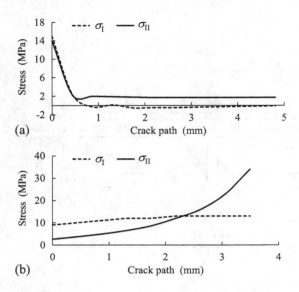

FIGURE 5.7 Stress profiles along the longitudinal crack path ahead of the crack tip just before; (a) damage onset and (b) crack starting advance.

crack initiation occurs under mixed-mode I+II instead of the intended pure mode II loading. The second relevant aspect relies on the alteration of the stress profiles between the two stages considered (Figure 5.7a and 5.7b), indicating that mode-mixity changes during damage propagation. This means that self-similar crack growth conditions are indeed not satisfied in the AFPB test.

The normalised R-curve was obtained for the AFPB following the same procedure described for the CS test. The curve plotted in Figure 5.8 reveals a monotonic rising trend depicting the alteration of mode-mixity as the crack grows. The discussed problems reveal that this test is not appropriate for pure mode II

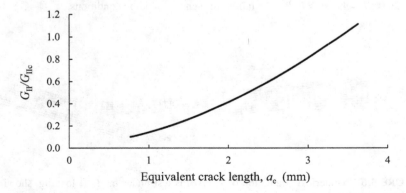

FIGURE 5.8 Normalised R-curve as a function of longitudinal crack extension, obtained for AFPB test.

fracture characterisation of cortical bone tissue since mixed-mode loading arises instead of pure mode II. In addition, the fact that mode-mixity alters markedly during crack propagation also invalidates its application regarding mixed-mode I+II fracture characterisation of cortical bone tissue.

5.3 NUMERICAL ANALYSIS OF THE END-LOADED SPLIT (ELS) TEST

The inadequacy of the previous tests to provide an accurate evaluation of mode II fracture energy of cortical bone led to the search for alternatives based on beam-type specimens. One of them is the miniaturised version of the end-loaded split (ELS) test [de Moura et al., 2010], which consists of a cantilever beam geometry, i.e., a pre-cracked clamped beam loaded at its free extremity (Figure 5.9). The application of loading leads to relative sliding between the specimen arms, thus inducing mode II shear loading at the crack extremity. The considered specimen dimensions (Figure 5.9) were selected according to the typical size possible to get in cortical bone tissue.

A refined finite element mesh used is shown in Figure 5.10. Clamping conditions were simulated by two rigid blocks tightening the specimen in the first step. It was verified [de Moura et al., 2010] that a tightening of 0.1 mm provides satisfactory measurements of mode II fracture energy (G_{IIc}) without overcoming the compressive strength of bone. Subsequently, a loading displacement is applied through the loading pin (Figure 5.10), considering very small increments (0.01% of total applied displacement) aiming to get smooth crack growth. The elastic properties are listed in Table 4.1. Typical values of local strength $\sigma_{u,II} = 51.6$ MPa [Turner et al., 2001] and mode II toughness $G_{IIc}=2.43$ N/mm [Feng et al., 2000] were used in the numerical analysis (Table 5.1). A trapezoidal law was considered with an arbitrary value for $\delta_{2,II} = 0.02$ mm (Figure 3.4).

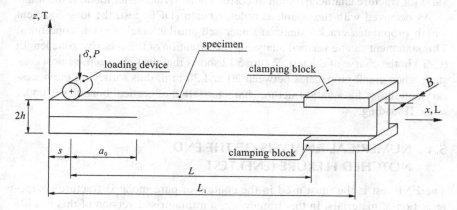

FIGURE 5.9 Schematic representation of the ELS test with $L_1 = 60$, $L = 48$, $2h = 6$, $a_0 = 20$, $B = 3.5$, $s = 4$; all dimensions in mm.

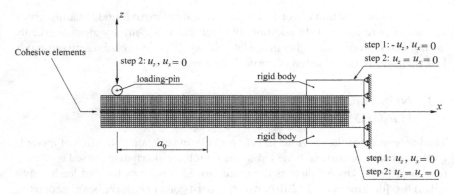

FIGURE 5.10   Finite element mesh used in the ELS test.

TABLE 5.1
Cohesive Properties of Bovine Bone

	$\sigma_{1,II}$ (MPa)	$\delta_{2,II}$ (mm)	$\delta_{3,II}$ (mm)	$\sigma_{3,II}$ (MPa)	G_{IIc} (N/mm)
Cortical bone	51.6	0.02	0.05	23.0	2.43

The numerical load–displacement curve and crack length evolution were recorded during the analysis to establish the $C = f(a)$ relation, to which a third-degree polynomial was adjusted (Figure 5.11a). After differentiation, the evolution of the strain energy release rate as a function of the crack length can be obtained by the Irwin–Kies relation (Eq. 3.5). Figure 5.11b presents a normalised R-curve revealing that the fracture energy (G_{IIc}) used as input is practically captured in the plateau region. From a theoretical perspective, it can be concluded that this test is valid for fracture characterisation of cortical bone tissue under mode II loading.

As occurred with the double cantilever beam (DCB) test, the long ligament length propitiates crack extension under self-similar crack growth conditions. This statement can be verified analysing the evolution of the cohesive zone length (CZL) in the course of the test. Figure 5.12 shows that the CZL keeps almost constant when crack propagates between 20 and 30 mm, thus satisfying the necessary conditions for a valid fracture characterisation of cortical bone tissue under mode II loading.

5.4   NUMERICAL ANALYSIS OF THE END-NOTCHED FLEXURE (ENF) TEST

The ENF test is the most used in the context of pure mode II fracture characterisation of materials. In this framework, a miniaturised version of this test [de Moura et al., 2010, F.A.M. Pereira et al., 2018] is analysed to assess its validity for cortical bone. The ENF test is a beam-type specimen with a pre-crack at one

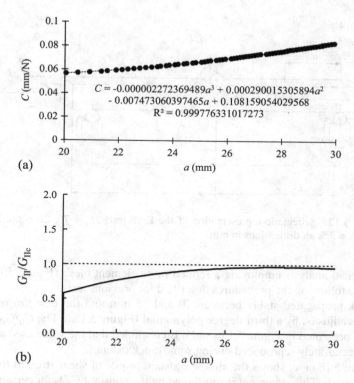

FIGURE 5.11 Results of ELS simulation: (a) $C = f(a)$ relationship adjusted by polynomial with third degree and (b) evolution of the strain energy release rate (G_{II}) normalised by the critical value G_{IIc} used as input in the simulation.

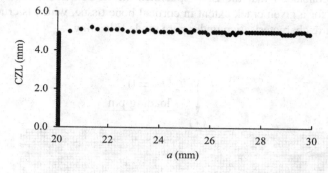

FIGURE 5.12 Evolution of the CZL as a function of crack growth in the ELS test.

of its extremities loaded in three-point bending (Figure 5.13). The applied loading induces longitudinal shear sliding at the crack tip, thus providing fracture characterisation under mode II loading. The elastic and fracture properties were the same as those used in the ELS test. Considering admissible cortical bone dimensions (Figure 5.13) for fracture characterisation in the TL fracture system,

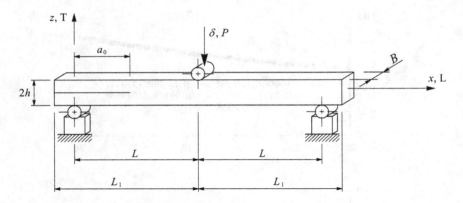

FIGURE 5.13 Schematic representation of the ENF test: $2L_1 = 70$, $2L = 60$, $2h = 6$, $a_0 = 20$, $B = 3.5$; all dimensions in mm.

a numerical analysis employing a refined finite element mesh (Figure 5.14) was executed following the procedures described for previous tests.

Crack propagated stably between 20 and 25 mm and the $C = f(a)$ relationship was adjusted by a third-degree polynomial (Figure 5.15a). The $G_{II}/G_{IIc} = f(a)$ curve is presented in Figure 5.15b and it is concluded that the value used as input (G_{IIc}) is accurately reproduced during some crack extent.

Figure 5.16 (a–c) shows the almost constant profile of shear stresses for some crack growth. This statement is reinforced by the constant CZL for certain crack propagation (Figure 5.16d), until the compressive stresses developing close to the central loading point start to exert their influence on the CZL-free development. It can be concluded that the ENF specimen allows self-similar crack growth conditions for a given crack extent in cortical bone tissue, which is crucial for a valid fracture characterisation under pure mode II loading.

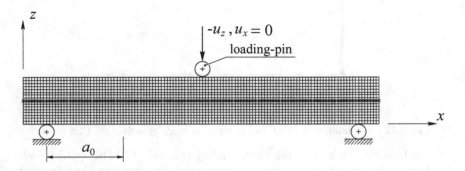

FIGURE 5.14 Finite element mesh used in the ENF test.

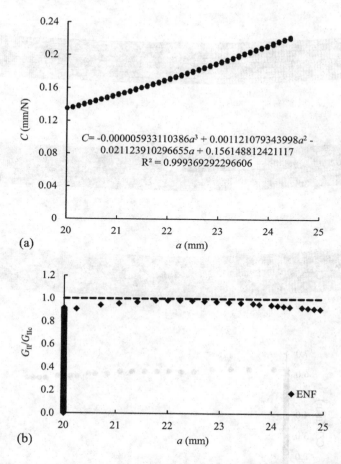

FIGURE 5.15 Results of ENF simulation: (a) $C = f(a)$ relationship adjusted by a third-degree polynomial and (b) evolution of the strain energy release rate (G_{II}) normalised by the critical value used as input (G_{IIc}) in the simulation.

5.5 ELS FRACTURE TESTS

5.5.1 EXPERIMENTAL TESTS

ELS tests were performed on bovine cortical bone tissue. Specimens' preparation procedure described for the DCB tests (Section 4.4) was followed in this case. Specimens were conceived in order to provide propagation in the TL fracture system (i.e., the normal to the crack plane is the tangential direction of mid-diaphysis and the crack propagation direction is the longitudinal direction of mid-diaphysis). Longitudinal grooves were also considered aiming to induce crack growth at the intended plane (Figure 5.17).

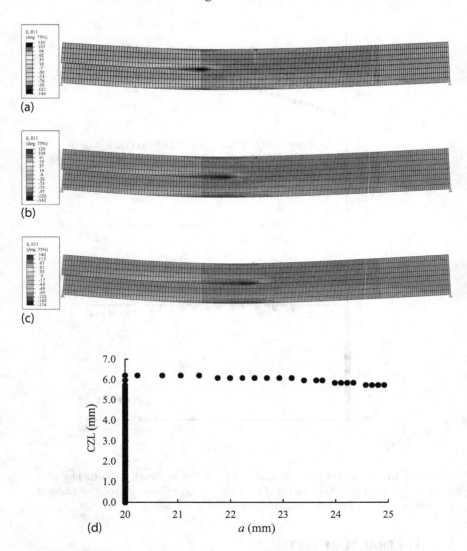

FIGURE 5.16 Evolution of (a–c) shear stresses during crack growth and (d) CZL as a function of crack length in the ENF test.

Fracture tests were performed under displacement control (0.5 mm/min) using a servo-electrical material testing system (MicroTester INSTRON 5848) with a 2 kN load cell, for an acquisition frequency of 5 Hz. During the test, the applied loading displacement (δ) and the resulting load (P) were registered. The fixture testing includes a linear guidance system (Figure 5.18), which allows horizontal translation of the clamping grip during the loading process. This solution avoids tensile stress development along the longitudinal direction, which would influence the measured results. As stated in Section 5.3, a tightening of 0.1 mm was

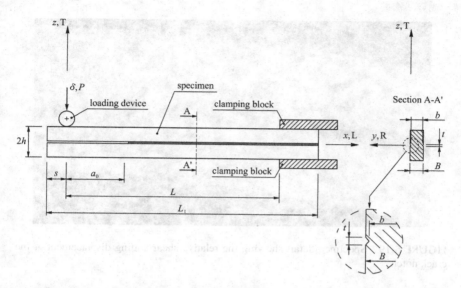

FIGURE 5.17 Schematic representation of the ELS test: $L_1 = 60$, $L = 50$, $s = 3$, $a_0 = 20$, $2h = 6$, $b = 2.5$, $B = 3.5$ and $t = 1$ (dimensions in mm).

applied. Two thin Teflon® films with a pellicle of lubricator between them were introduced in the pre-crack region (Figure 5.18) aiming to minimise the friction effects.

Figure 5.19 shows the detail of crack surfaces shear sliding at the notch tip during propagation, which reveals the existence of mode II loading. It can also be observed that the crack-tip position is not easily identifiable with the required accuracy. Consequently, the application of classical data reduction schemes based

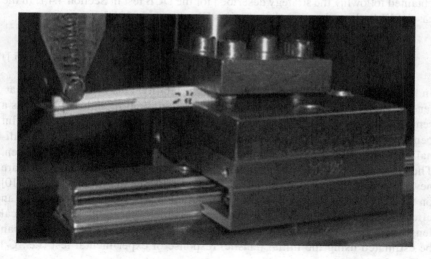

FIGURE 5.18 Testing setup for the ELS test.

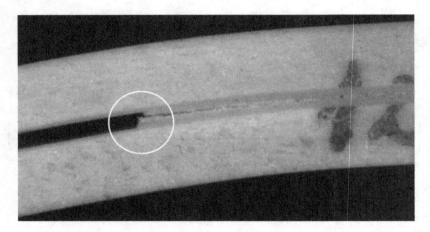

FIGURE 5.19 Specimen detail showing the relative shear sliding displacement at the crack notch.

on crack length (a) monitoring during propagation can lead to inaccurate estimations of fracture energy, due to errors committed on crack length measurements. In order to solve this difficulty, an equivalent crack length-based method was developed for the ELS test.

5.5.2 COMPLIANCE-BASED BEAM METHOD (CBBM)
APPLIED TO THE ELS TEST

The relationship between specimen compliance (C) and crack length (a) is obtained following the strategy described for the DCB test in Section 4.4.1. In the case of ELS, the following relation arises [Pereira et al., 2011]

$$C - \frac{3a^3}{2Bh^3E_L} = \frac{L^3}{2Bh^3E_L} + \frac{3L}{5BhG_{LT}} \tag{5.1}$$

In the ELS tests, there are two sources of variability. One of them is the scatter of the elastic properties, namely on the longitudinal modulus, which has a remarkable influence on the results. The solution was to perform three-point bending tests on all the specimens before executing the notch and longitudinal grooves aiming to determine the longitudinal modulus of each specimen. The other source of inconsistency is related to clamping conditions, which are never perfect and revealed to have a relevant influence [de Moura et al., 2010] on measured results. A valid strategy to include their effects is considering an effective specimen length (L_{ef} instead of L), which represents the theoretical length that specimens should have to satisfy Eq. (5.1). This parameter (L_{ef}) can be estimated using the initial (elastic) response of experimental test (i.e., C_0) in Eq. (5.1),

$$C_0 - \frac{3a_0^3}{2Bh^3 E_L} = \frac{L_{ef}^3}{2Bh^3 E_L} + \frac{3L_{ef}}{5BhG_{LT}} \tag{5.2}$$

By combining Eqs. (5.1) and (5.2), the equivalent crack length (instead of a) during propagation becomes

$$a_e = \left[(C - C_0)\frac{2Bh^3 E_L}{3} + a_0^3 \right]^{\frac{1}{3}} \tag{5.3}$$

not depending on parameters L_{ef} and G_{LT}. The evolution of the strain energy release rate in mode II (G_{II}) as a function of the equivalent crack length (a_e) can be obtained by combining Eq. (4.9) for mode II, with Eqs. (5.1) and (5.3), yielding

$$G_{II} = \frac{9P^2 a_e^2}{4bBh^3 E_L} \tag{5.4}$$

Following this methodology, the mode II R-curve is obtained as a function of a_e and the critical fracture energy G_{IIc} is captured from its plateau. The method only requires the previous measurement of E_L as well as the load–displacement data obtained during the experimental test. Hence, the problem associated with crack length monitoring is solved, since the equivalent crack length became a calculated parameter instead of a measured one. Additionally, this procedure allows accounting indirectly for a non-negligible fracture process zone (FPZ). In fact, the FPZ influences specimen compliance that is used to obtain the R-curve.

The experimental tests were performed under the same conditions and followed the same procedures considered in the DCB tests. The load–displacement values of the valid results are presented in Figure 5.20, exhibiting consistency with each other. The corresponding R-curves are presented in Figure 5.21, thus revealing the typical profile constituted by an initial rising trend representative of

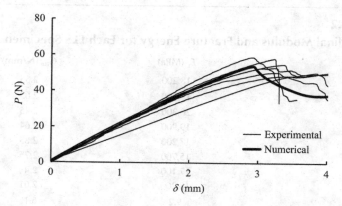

FIGURE 5.20   Load–displacement curves of the quasi-static ELS tests.

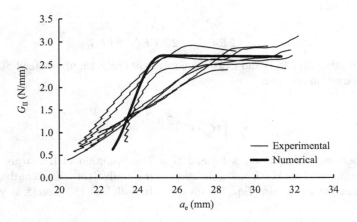

FIGURE 5.21   *R*-curves of the quasi-static ELS tests.

the FPZ development followed by a plateau region demonstrative of the self-similar crack growth. The values of the plateau define the fracture energy under mode II loading and point to an average of $G_{IIc} = 2.61$ N/mm (Table 5.2). This value was used as input in a cohesive zone analysis (Figure 5.10) considering the nominal specimen dimensions (Figure 5.17), the cohesive parameters presented in Section 5.3 and the average elastic longitudinal modulus of this set of specimens (Table 5.2). The numerical load–displacement and respective *R*-curves were included in Figures 5.20 and 5.21. It can be verified that good reproducibility values of the experimental trends were obtained in both cases, which validates the experimental procedure and the ELS test in the context of mode II fracture characterisation of cortical bone tissue.

TABLE 5.2

Longitudinal Modulus and Fracture Energy for Each ELS Specimen

Specimen	E_L (MPa)	G_{IIc} (N/mm)
1	18,200	2.55
2	19,200	2.65
3	20,300	2.45
4	19,900	2.64
5	17,200	2.85
6	15,700	2.75
7	17,100	2.4
Average	18,200	2.61
CoV (%)	9.2	6.1

5.6 ENF FRACTURE TESTS

Mode II fracture characterisation of bovine cortical bone tissue in the TL fracture system was performed employing the ENF test (Figure 5.22). Longitudinal grooves were considered aiming to get propagation along the specimen midplane. The quasi-static tests were performed imposing a loading displacement rate of 0.1 mm/min using a servo-electrical material testing system (MicroTester INSTRON 5848) with a 2 kN load cell for an acquisition frequency of 5 Hz. In order to minimise spurious friction effects, two Teflon® films with a pellicle of lubricant between them were introduced in the pre-crack region (Figure 5.23).

Figure 5.24 (Detail A) reveals the relative shear displacement at the notch tip proving the existence of shear sliding characteristic of mode II loading. It is also clear that the crack-tip position is not easily identified with accuracy in the ENF test (Figure 5.24 – Detail B). In fact, under pure mode II loading, cracks tend to

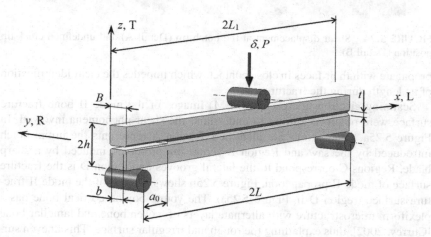

FIGURE 5.22 Schematic representation of the ENF test: $2L_1 = 65$; $2L = 60$; $2h = 6$; $t = 1$; $B = 3.5$; $b = 2.5$; $a_0 = 20$ (all dimensions in mm).

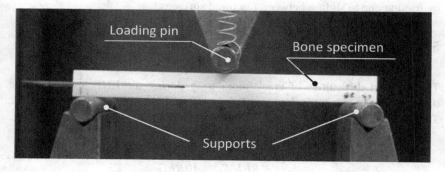

FIGURE 5.23 Testing setup for the ENF test.

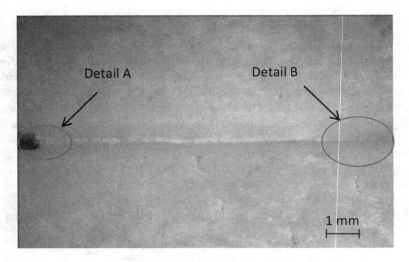

FIGURE 5.24   Shear displacement at the notch tip (Detail A) and undefined crack-tip position (Detail B).

propagate with their faces in close contact, which impedes the clear identification of its length during the fracture test.

Scanning electron microscopy (SEM) images of the mode II bone fracture surface were obtained aiming to understand the shear phenomena involved. In Figure 5.25a, four regions are identified. Region A represents the initial notch introduced by the saw and Region B shows the pre-crack induced by a sharp blade. Regions C correspond to the lateral grooves and region D is the fracture surface of mode II propagation. Figure 5.25b shows a detail of the mode II fracture surface (region D in Figure 5.25a). The young bovine cortical bone has a plexiform microstructure with alternate layers of woven bone and lamellar bone [Currey, 2002], thus explaining the rough and irregular surface. This uneven surface is responsible for the increase of fracture energy during crack propagation under mode II loading by several damage mechanisms: micro-crack development, crack deflection in crack path and surface roughness that dissipates energy by friction due to sliding between fractured surfaces.

5.6.1   Compliance-Based Beam Method (CBBM) Applied to the ENF Test

The referred difficulties of crack monitoring during the ENF test led to the development of an equivalent crack length-based procedure. Considering the Timoshenko beam theory, the $C = f(a)$ relationship writes [Dourado et al., 2013],

$$C = \frac{3a^3 + 2L^3}{8Bh^3 E_L} + \frac{3L}{10Bh\,G_{LT}} \qquad (5.5)$$

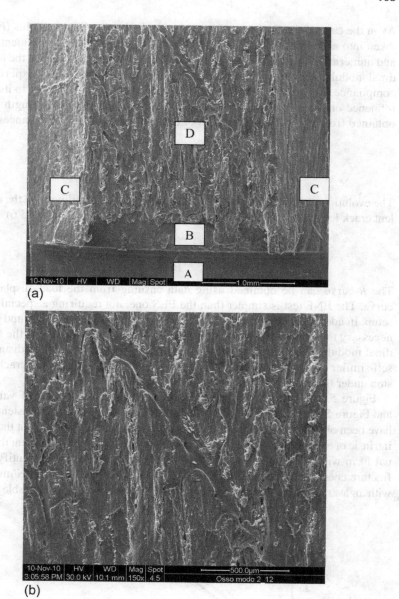

FIGURE 5.25 (a) Fracture surface: A – initial notch; B – pre-crack using a blade; C – lateral grooves; D – mode II fracture surface; (b) detail of fracture surface of region D.

As in the case of the DCB test, the scatter on the longitudinal modulus (E_L) was taken into account following an inverse procedure combining experimental data and numerical analysis. The procedure is based on iteratively altering the longitudinal modulus (E_L) in the numerical analysis aiming to fit the initial experimental compliance. A typical value of G_{LT} (Table 4.1) was considered owing to its minor influence on the measured fracture energy. The equivalent crack length can be obtained from Eq. (5.5) as a function of the current specimen compliance (C)

$$a_e = \left[\left(C - \frac{3L}{10 G_{LT} Bh} \right) \frac{8 E_L B h^3}{3} - \frac{2L^3}{3} \right]^{\frac{1}{3}} \tag{5.6}$$

The evolution of strain energy release rate under mode II loading with the equivalent crack length can be obtained by combining Eqs. (4.1), (5.5) and (5.6)

$$G_{II} = \frac{9 P^2 a_e^2}{16 b B h^3 E_L} \tag{5.7}$$

The R-curve can be obtained using data ensuing from the load–displacement curve. The ENF test is simpler than the ELS one, not requiring a special testing setup. In addition, the variability induced by clamping does not arise and it is not necessary to perform preliminary three-point bending tests to assess the longitudinal modulus. The only disadvantage of the ENF regards its lesser distance for self-similar crack growth, but it was proved in Section 5.4 that some crack extension under these optimal conditions is still possible.

Figure 5.26 shows the experimental load–displacement curves of valid tests and Figure 5.27 the respective R-curves. It can be concluded that consistent results have been obtained in this set of samples, especially taking into account the scatter intrinsic of a natural material, as is the case of bone. The R-curves present the habitual form with an initial rising trend followed by a plateau region identifying the fracture energy under mode II loading. The values are in the 1.5–2.5 N/mm range with an average of 2.1 N/mm and a coefficient of variation of 17.3% (Table 5.3).

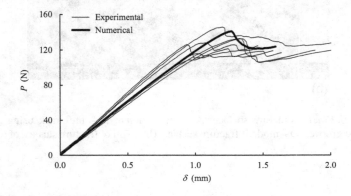

FIGURE 5.26   Load–displacement curves of the quasi-static ENF tests.

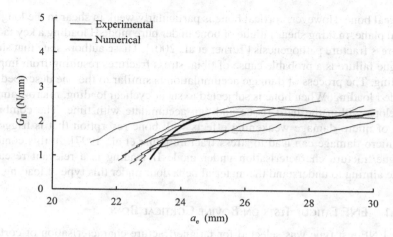

FIGURE 5.27 *R*-curves of the quasi-static ENF tests.

TABLE 5.3
Longitudinal Modulus and Fracture Energy for Each ENF Specimen

Specimen	E_L (MPa)	G_{IIc} (N/mm)
1	16,900	2.5
2	15,800	1.8
3	18,900	1.9
4	18,700	2.4
5	14,800	2.3
6	15,300	1.5
7	15,400	2.1
Average	16,500	2.1
CoV (%)	10.1	17.3

The average values of Table 5.3 were used as input in a finite element analysis using cohesive zone modelling. The ensuing numerical load–displacement and *R*-curves were included in Figures 5.26 and 5.27, respectively. It can be concluded that they are representative of the observed experimental trends, which serves to validate the ENF test and all the procedures as a valid option regarding mode II fracture characterisation of cortical bone tissue.

5.7 FATIGUE/FRACTURE CHARACTERISATION UNDER MODE II LOADING

Fatigue under shear stress is usually caused by repetitive loading torsion resulting from demanding physical activities, as is the case of sports or dancing practice. Torsional loading induces both transverse and longitudinal shear stresses in the cortical bone. However, cortical bone is particularly weak in shear in the longitudinal plane, making shear fatigue of bone under pure mode II loading a key factor in stress fracture pathogenesis [Turner et al., 2001]. These authors state that shear fatigue failure is a probable cause of tibial stress fractures resulting from impact loading. The process of damage accumulation is similar to the one described for mode I loading. When bone is subjected to shear cyclical loading, micro-damage develops within the hard tissue and can accumulate with time. The combination of micro-damage weakening effects with bone resorption that is triggered by micro-damage can lead to stress fracture [Burr et al., 1997]. In this context, fatigue/fracture characterisation under mode II loading is a relevant research topic aiming to understand the material behaviour under this type of loading.

5.7.1 ENF FATIGUE TESTS ON BOVINE CORTICAL BONE

The ENF test type was selected for fatigue/fracture characterisation of cortical bone tissue under pure mode II loading taking into consideration its simplicity and adequacy observed for quasi-static fracture characterisation. A preliminary quasi-static test inducing a quite small crack growth was performed (Figure 5.28) to get an accurate estimation of the ultimate load (P_u) and fracture energy (G_{IIc})

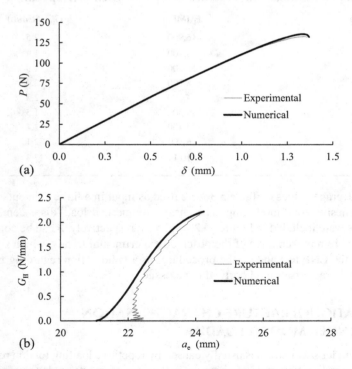

(a)

(b)

FIGURE 5.28 Experimental and numerical: (a) load–displacement curves and (b) *R*-curves of a preliminary quasi-static ENF test.

for each specimen, thus diminishing the effect of scatter. These values were used to define individually the maximum load of the fatigue test ($P_{max}=P_u/2$) and G_{IIc}, which is a crucial parameter in the post-processing analysis of fatigue results employing the modified Paris law (Eq. 3.45). A numerical analysis of the quasi-static test was also carried out to confirm the correct evaluation of P_u and G_{IIc}. The good agreement between the numerical and experimental curves reveals that these parameters were well captured, i.e., when P_u is attained, a plateau develops in the numerical R-curve defining the fracture energy G_{IIc} that is in agreement with the experimental value (Figure 5.28). The pronounced variations in the early stage of the experimental R-curve are due to small variations in compliance that occur at the beginning of the experimental test.

Fatigue tests were performed immediately after the quasi-test test considering loading control, a load ratio in a cycle $R=P_{min}/P_{max}=0.1$ and a frequency of 2 Hz. Specimens were continuously irrigated in the course of the test guaranteeing their hydration, thus diminishing premature unwanted failures. The evolution of the specimen compliance C as a function of the number of cycles N is registered. The equivalent crack length (a_e) and the corresponding strain energy release rate under mode II loading (G_{II}) are obtained by Eqs. (5.6) and (5.7), respectively. The modified Paris law under mode II loading becomes

$$\frac{dA_e}{dN} = C_{1,II}\left(\frac{\Delta G_{II}}{G_{IIc}}\right)^{C_{2,II}} = C_{1,II}\left[\frac{G_{II,max}\left(1-R\right)^2}{G_{IIc}}\right]^{C_{2,II}} \tag{5.8}$$

where ΔG_{II} and $G_{II,max}$ are the variation and maximum values of the mode II strain energy release rate in a cycle, respectively, G_{IIc} is the mode II fracture energy and $C_{1,II}$, $C_{2,II}$ are the Paris law coefficients for mode II loading.

Figure 5.29 reveals a typical example of the post-processing analysis. The curve showing the compliance versus the number of cycles (Figure 5.29a) enables the achievement of the equivalent crack length evolution as a function of the number of cycles (Figure 5.29b) using Eq. (5.6). Subsequently, the evolution of the variation of the normalized strain energy release rate in a cycle ($\Delta G_{II}/G_{IIc}$) with the number of cycles is easily obtained (Figure 5.29c) applying Eq. (5.7). These three curves reveal a moderate increase up to 110,000 cycles mimicking stable damage propagation. From this point, a second stage with higher growth rate occurs representing Region III of the fatigue curve (Figure 3.1). The coefficients of the Paris law are obtained from the region of stable crack propagation (in the range of 50,000–110,000 cycles). The growth rate of damaged area (dA_e/dN) as a function of the energy ratio ($\Delta G_{II}/G_{IIc}$) is plotted in Figure 5.29d using a bi-logarithmic representation for the stable crack propagation region. Although some scatter can be observed, a rising tendency is visible reflecting the expected damage rate increase with the number of cycles.

The evolution of normalised compliance with the number of cycles corresponding to all valid tests is grouped in Figure 5.30. The normalisation by the specimen dimensions aims to minimize scatter on initial specimen compliance. It

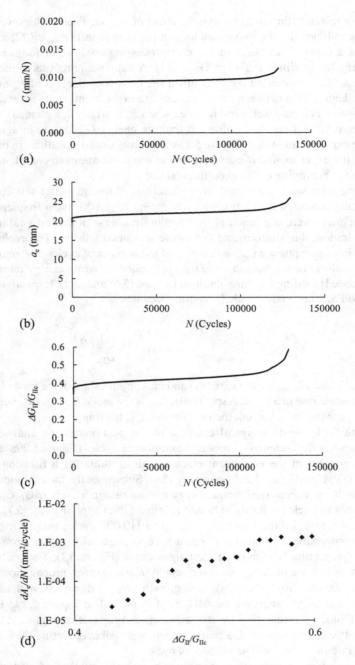

(a)

(b)

(c)

(d)

FIGURE 5.29 Evolution of (a) specimen compliance; (b) equivalent crack length; (c) variation of normalised strain energy release rate under mode II loading as function of number of cycles; (d) damaged area growth rate in function of energy ratio.

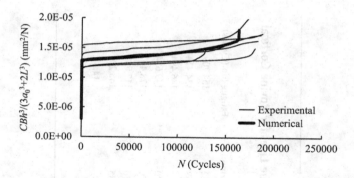

FIGURE 5.30 Normalised compliance versus number of cycles of valid results obtained for bovine cortical bone tissue.

can be observed that the majority of the specimens failed in the range of 120,000–180,000 cycles. The power law adjusted to all results in Figure 5.31 provides the coefficients of the modified Paris law ($C_1 = 0.0005$ mm²/cycle, $C_2 = 2.3073$), which defines the stable damage growth rate of this ensemble of bovine bone samples under mode II loading. Table 5.4 summarises the specimen dimensions and properties besides the corresponding fatigue lives.

A numerical analysis was performed for the ENF fatigue tests. The coefficients of the modified Paris law were considered, together with the average dimensions and material properties (Table 5.4). The ensuing numerical normalised compliance versus the number of cycles curve was included in Figure 5.30, for comparison with the experimental ones. The numerical curve reveals a continuously rising trend from the beginning, mimicking gradual material degradation as a function of the number of cycles (see Eq. 3.55). The experimental curves are generally flatter, revealing slighter rising trends until abrupt failure. This different behaviour is probably dictated by fatigue threshold, which was not determined experimentally and consequently not addressed in this numerical model. Anyway, it can be affirmed that the numerical model reproduces the overall experimental trend and the fatigue life defined by the abrupt increase of slope of the numerical curve.

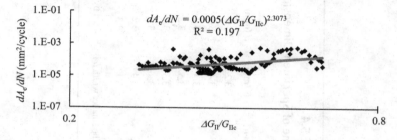

FIGURE 5.31 Bi-logarithmic representation of fatigue damage growth rate (dA_e/dN) versus $\Delta G_{II}/G_{IIc}$ for a set of bovine bone specimens.

TABLE 5.4

Resume of Specimen Dimensions, Properties, Maximum Loads, Fracture Properties and Fatigue Lives for Bovine Cortical Bone

Specimen	B (mm)	h (mm)	a_0 (mm)	L (mm)	E_L (MPa)	P_{max} (N)	σ_{ult} (MPa)	G_{IIc} (N/mm)	Fatigue life (Cycles)
1	3.2	3.3	21.6	30	10,372	65	57	1.72	154,709
2	3.4	3.1	21.6	30	10,418	68	61	1.68	134,414
3	3.4	3.2	20.0	30	12,052	71	62	2.00	136,494
4	3.5	3.2	19.7	30	12,685	68	43	2.20	149,624
5	3.3	3.1	19.7	30	9,267	74	49	1.79	178,457
6	3.4	3.0	20.2	30	10,591	75	40	1.70	117,738
Average	3.4	3.2	20.5	30	10,898	70	52.0	1.85	145,239
CoV (%)	3.1	3.3	4.4	0.0	11.5	5.5	18.0	11.3	14.3

Note: The smaller width b is obtained by subtracting 1 mm from B (Figure 5.22).

5.8 SUMMARY

The mode II quasi-static and fatigue/fracture characterisation of cortical bone tissue is addressed in this chapter. An initial numerical procedure was performed on typical mode II fracture tests used in the context of cortical bone tissue. It was concluded that the end-loaded split and the end-notched flexure tests were both appropriate to determine the fracture energy under mode II loading of hydrated cortical bone, and they were used for quasi-static procedures. In both cases, equivalent crack length-based methodologies were developed in order to avoid non-rigorous crack length monitoring in the course of the fracture tests. The fracture energies under pure mode II loading obtained from the two types of fracture tests can be considered coherent taking into consideration the scatter inherent to a natural material. Fatigue/fracture studies were performed considering the end-notched flexure tests owing to their simpler setup. The coefficients of the modified Paris law for pure mode II loading and the fatigue lives were obtained. Numerical analysis aiming to validate the approaches employed in the quasi-static and fatigue/fracture analyses were performed. Overall, a good representation of the experimental trends has been achieved.

6 Mixed-Mode I+II Fracture Characterisation

Fracture characterisation of cortical bone tissue under pure modes (I and II) is important for specific and particular cases of loading. However, under general loading, fracture conditions involving simultaneously mode I and II (mixed-mode I+II) will prevail. In general, cracks formed and initiated in bone are subjected to mixed-mode tensile-shear conditions. This is essentially promoted by the non-symmetric geometry and irregular shape of bone, the complexity of the mechanical multiaxial loads induced by common daily activities, the orientation of cracks relative to the applied loads and the bone anisotropy that defines directions prone to failure. Effectively, the marked anisotropy induced by the alignment of osteons along the axis of long bones delineates regions prone to crack propagation (i.e., paths). Consequently, cracks can initiate and propagate under mixed-mode conditions since they are confined and obliged to grow in pre-established regions, e.g., predominantly on the direction of the osteons along outermost lamellae, characterised by lower fracture energy. Accordingly, in practice, the fracture properties under mode I, mode II and the corresponding fracture envelope influence the process of initiation and propagation of a macro-crack from the tip of pre-existing small cracks in bone. The circumstance that the fracture toughness can vary as a function of loading mode highlights the need to characterise the fracture resistance of bone under more realistic mixed-mode conditions. Therefore, the definition of a cortical bone fracture criterion in the mode I versus mode II space, usually labelled as the fracture envelope, is a fundamental task.

With this aim, specific tests for bone fracture characterisation under mixed-mode I+II loading have been proposed. George and Vashishth [2006] studied the combined effect of axial–torsional fatigue loading on fracture considering cylindrical dumbbell specimens (Figure 2.6a) with reduced gauge section machined from medial and lateral cortices of 19 human male donor tibiae. They conducted fatigue tests under physiologically relevant loading involving simultaneous application of axial and torsional loading to produce previously reported *in vivo* shear/normal stress ratios.

Zimmermann et al. [2009, 2010] proposed the asymmetric four-point bending (AFPB) test, which provides several combinations of shear force and bending moment acting at the crack tip (Figure 5.5), thus allowing characterisation under different mixed-mode I+II loading. However, the numerical analyses described in Section 5.2 reveal that a remarkable alteration of the stress profiles takes place

DOI: 10.1201/9781003375081-6

during propagation, meaning that the mode ratio is not constant during crack growth. Consequently, self-similar crack growth conditions are not fulfilled in the AFPB test, making it unsuitable for a valid mixed-mode I+II fracture characterisation of cortical bone tissue.

Olvera et al. [2012] used the double-cleavage drilled compression (DCDC) test geometry in the context of mixed-mode I+II fracture characterisation of cortical bone tissue. This test has been applied to other materials [He et al., 1995; Lardner et al., 2001] and consists of a parallelepipedic column containing a longitudinal crack with a circular hole drilled through its centre and submitted to axial compression loading (Figure 6.1). Due to the presence of the hole of radius R, tensile and shear stresses are generated in the vicinity of the crack tip inducing mixed-mode I+II loading. The DCDC test allows mixed-mode I+II fracture characterisation for the range $0° \leq \psi \leq 64°$, where the phase angle ψ is given by

$$\psi = \text{arctg}\,(K_{II}/K_{I}) \tag{6.1}$$

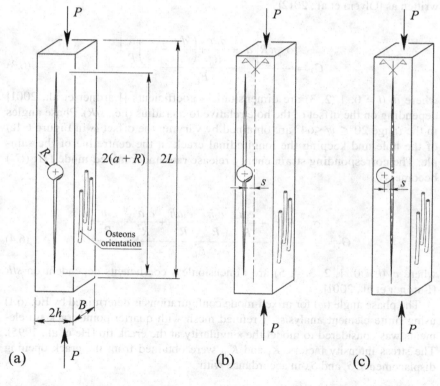

FIGURE 6.1 The DCDC test geometry; (a) pure mode I loading; (b) mixed-mode I+II for phase angles $0 \leq \psi \leq 20°$; (c) mixed-mode I+II for phase angles $20° \leq \psi \leq 64°$. Bone specimen dimensions (in mm) are: $2L = 39.8$–41.4, $2h = 4.0$–4.3, $B = 2.9$-4.5, $R = 0.50$–0.75, $13.4 \leq 2(a+R) \leq 18.0$.

with K_I and K_{II} being the mode I and mode II stress intensity factors, respectively. Three different cases can be considered depending on the locations of the longitudinal crack and the hole. The pure mode I condition ($\psi = 0°$) arises when the hole and the crack are aligned with the centreline of the sample (Figure 6.1a). The mode I strain energy release rate (G_I) can be given in terms of the applied stress (σ_{ap}) [Olvera et al., 2012],

$$G_I = \frac{\sigma_{ap}^2 \pi R \left[\dfrac{h}{R} + \left(\dfrac{0.235h}{R} - 0.259 \right) \dfrac{a}{R} \right]^{-2}}{E_L'} \qquad (6.2)$$

where E_L' is the appropriate elastic modulus given by the longitudinal Young's modulus E_L for plane stress or by $E_L/(1-v_{LT})$ for plane strain, being v_{LT} the Poisson's ratio. The mixed-mode I+II conditions ($0° \le \psi \le 20°$) occur at the crack tip, when the hole and the crack are offset from the centreline of the sample (distance s in Figure 6.1b). The strain energy release rate under mixed-mode I+II (G_T) can be written as [Olvera et al., 2012]

$$G_T = \frac{\sigma_{ap}^2 \pi R \left[d_0 + \dfrac{d_1 a}{R} + \left(\dfrac{d_2 h}{R} - d_3 \right) \dfrac{a}{R} \right]^{-2}}{E_L'} \qquad (6.3)$$

where d_i ($i = 0, 1, 2, 3$) are dimensionless coefficients [Lardner et al., 2001] depending on the offset of the hole relative to its radius (i.e., s/R). Phase angles in the range $20° \le \psi \le 64°$ are obtained by varying the offset (s in Figure 6.1c) of the hole and keeping the longitudinal crack in the centreline of the sample. The corresponding strain energy release rate under mixed-mode I+II (G_T) becomes

$$G_T = \frac{\sigma_{ap}^2 \pi R \left[c_0 + \dfrac{c_1 a}{R} + \dfrac{c_2 h}{R} + \dfrac{c_3 a h}{R^2} + \dfrac{c_4 a^2}{R^2} + \dfrac{c_5 h^2}{R^2} \right]^{-2}}{E_L'} \qquad (6.4)$$

where c_i ($i = 0, 1, 2, 3, 4, 5$) are dimensionless coefficients dependent on s/R [Lardner et al., 2001].

The phase angle (ψ) for mixed-mode configurations is determined by Eq. (6.1) using finite element analysis. A refined mesh with quarter-point crack tip elements was considered to model the singularity at the crack tip [He et al., 1995]. The stress intensity factors, K_I and K_{II}, were obtained from the crack opening displacements, δ_x and δ_y, in accordance with

$$\left(K_I, K_{II} \right) = \frac{E_L' \pi^{1/2}}{4\sqrt{2}} \lim_{r \to 0} \left(\frac{\delta_y}{r^{1/2}}, \frac{\delta_x}{r^{1/2}} \right) \qquad (6.5)$$

where r is the distance from the crack tip in polar coordinates. This test has some drawbacks regarding mixed-mode I+II fracture characterisation of anisotropic and heterogeneous materials. The first aspect addresses the assumption that the two cracks generated at each crown of the hole propagate symmetrically along the axial direction of the sample as the loading compression increases. This rarely occurs due to inevitable small geometric misalignments and internal material heterogeneity, characteristic of a natural material as is the case of bone. In addition, the developed analysis involving Eqs. (6.1–6.5) is valid for brittle materials. In fact, the stress intensity factor K characterises the local distribution of stress and displacement in the vicinity of a sharp crack in a linear elastic solid. However, as previously discussed, bone is a quasi-brittle material developing a non-negligible fracture process zone ahead of the crack tip owing to several damage mechanisms. These aspects limit the applicability of this test regarding accurate mixed-mode I+II fracture characterisation of cortical bone tissue.

Aliha and Mousavi, [2020] proposed the sub-sized short bend beam configuration (Figure 6.2) for the study of mixed-mode I+II bone fracture. This test consists of a symmetric three-point bend loading on a short beam (SB) specimen containing an inclined edge crack with length a created in the middle of the sample. Owing to its small dimensions, the SB specimen is suitable to be employed in cases where a limited amount of raw material is available for the preparation of the test sample. The whole range of mode-mixity can be achieved by changing three geometrical and loading parameters (i.e., $a/2h$, $S/2h$ and α, see Figure 6.2), being the crack inclination angle α the most relevant in changing the mode-mixity. The mode I and mode II stress intensity factors in the SB specimen are given by

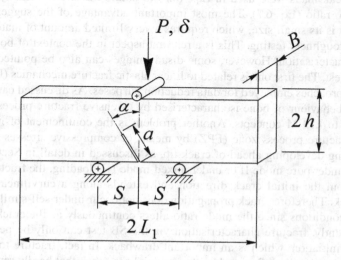

FIGURE 6.2 Schematic representation of the SB test. Specimen dimensions (in mm) are $2L_1 = 36$, $2S = 12$, $2h = 12$, $B = 4$, $a_0 = 6$.

$$K_{\mathrm{I}} = \frac{P}{2hB}\sqrt{\pi a}\, f_{\mathrm{I}}\!\left(\frac{a}{2h}, \frac{S}{2h}, \alpha\right)$$

$$K_{\mathrm{II}} = \frac{P}{2hB}\sqrt{\pi a}\, f_{\mathrm{II}}\!\left(\frac{a}{2h}, \frac{S}{2h}, \alpha\right)$$

(6.6)

where f_{I} and f_{II} are the modes I and II geometry factors, respectively, that are functions of crack length ratio ($a/2h$), bottom loading span ratio ($S/2h$) and crack inclination angle (α). These two geometry factors are independent of the material type and only depend on the geometry and loading conditions of the test specimen. Consequently, they were determined by performing finite element analyses and considering an elastic and homogeneous medium for any desired mixed-mode test configuration. The stress intensity factors for each geometry and loading condition (i.e., $a/2h$, $S/2h$ and α) are obtained from the finite element analyses and the corresponding values of geometry factors (f_{I} and f_{II}) can be determined from Eq. (6.6). Subsequently, the mode-mixity can be achieved from

$$M^{\mathrm{e}} = \frac{2}{\pi}\mathrm{arctg}\!\left(\frac{K_{\mathrm{I}}}{K_{\mathrm{II}}}\right)$$

(6.7)

It was verified that pure mode I and II loading conditions arise for $\alpha = 0°$ and for $35° \leq \alpha \leq 55°$ (depending on $a/2h$, $S/2h$ values), respectively.

The authors performed experimental tests considering specimens of bovine cortical bone whose length is oriented parallel to the longitudinal axis of it, with the dimensions shown in Figure 6.2. Five crack inclination angles were considered: 0° (pure mode I), 15°, 26°, 33° and 39° (pure mode II). The corresponding critical peak loads were used in Eqs. (6.6) to obtain the stress intensity factors and mode ratio (Eq. 6.7). The most important advantage of the suggested SB specimen is its small size, which requires a very limited amount of material for fracture toughness testing. This is a relevant aspect in the context of bone fracture characterisation. However, some disadvantages can also be pointed to this fracture test. The first one is related to linear elastic fracture mechanics (LEFM)-based approaches employed for data reduction purposes. As discussed earlier, the fracture behaviour of bone is characterised by extensive fracture process zones unsuited to LEFM concepts. Another problem is the confinement of non-negligible fracture process zone (FPZ) by means of compressive stresses induced by bending developing ahead of crack tip, as discussed in detail in Section 4.2. Finally, under pure mode II or under mixed-mode I+II loading, the fracture path kinks from the initial crack direction and extends along a curvilinear trajectory crack. Therefore, crack propagation does not occur under self-similar crack growth conditions since the mode ratio alters continuously as the crack grows. Consequently, fracture characterisation via the SB test can only be performed at crack initiation, which is an important drawback. In fact, fracture toughness values are markedly influenced by the artificial pre-crack that hardly reproduces rigorously a real crack and by small imperfections inherent to a natural and quite inhomogeneous material. To solve these shortcomings, obtaining the R-curves is important as these spurious effects can be overcome.

The tests described here have provided valuable insight into the role of various parameters in bone fracture behaviour under mixed-mode I+II loading. However, as discussed in this section, all of them reveal several deficiencies concerning suitable mixed-mode I+II fracture characterisation of bone. In this context, two alternative fracture tests are investigated and discussed in the following sections.

6.1 NUMERICAL ANALYSIS OF THE SINGLE-LEG BENDING (SLB) TEST

The SLB test is quite similar to the end-notched flexure (ENF) test employed for mode II fracture characterisation of bone and described in Section 5.6. As in the ENF case, the test is quite simple since it consists of a three-point-bend loading on a beam specimen with a pre-crack. The difference is on the lower specimen arm in the region of the pre-crack, which is shorter (Figure 6.3) and not loaded aiming to induce mixed-mode I+II loading. Indeed, the applied loading induces simultaneous longitudinal shear sliding and opening displacements at the crack tip, thus enabling fracture characterisation under mode I+II loading.

A preliminary finite element analysis of the miniaturised version of the SLB test (Figure 6.4) considering the nominal dimensions presented in Figure 6.3 was

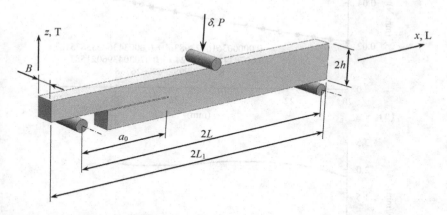

FIGURE 6.3 Schematic representation of the SLB test. Nominal dimensions are (in mm): $2L_1 = 65$, $2L = 60$, $2h = 6$, $a_0 = 20$, $B = 3.5$.

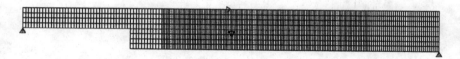

FIGURE 6.4 Finite element mesh used in the SLB test.

performed aiming to verify the adequacy of the test regarding bone fracture characterisation under mixed-mode I+II loading.

The simulations were performed considering the elastic properties of Table 4.1, the fracture energies used in the validation of the pure mode fracture tests (G_{Ic} = 1.77 N/mm and G_{IIc} = 2.43 N/mm) and the linear energetic criterion (Eq. 3.20 with γ = 1). Stable crack growth was obtained in the range $20 \leq a \leq 28$ mm enabling to adjust a third-degree polynomial to the $C = f(a)$ relationship (Figure 6.5a). After differentiation, the Irwin–Kies relation (Eq. 3.5) is used to obtain the evolution of the total strain energy release rate (G_T) as a function of the crack length (Figure 6.5b).

The value obtained during propagation points to $G_T \approx 2.0$ N/mm. Additionally, it is known that the SLB specimen with arms of equal thickness provides a constant mode-mixity $G_{II}/G_T \approx 0.43$ [Moreira et al., 2020]. Substituting this relation into $G_T = G_I + G_{II}$ gives rise to G_I = 1.14 N/mm and G_{II} = 0.86 N/mm. These energy components were included in the plot of G_I versus G_{II} (Figure 6.6) considering the linear energetic criterion (Eq. 3.20 with γ = 1). It can be verified that the SLB value is in close agreement with the used linear energetic criterion, which

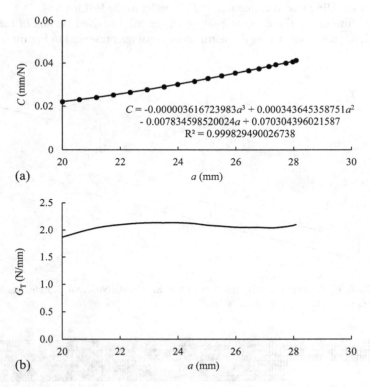

(a)

$$C = -0.000003616723983a^3 + 0.000343645358751a^2 - 0.007834598520024a + 0.070304396021587$$
$$R^2 = 0.999829490026738$$

(b)

FIGURE 6.5 Results of SLB simulation: (a) $C = f(a)$ relationship adjusted by polynomial with third degree and (b) evolution of the total strain energy release rate (G_T).

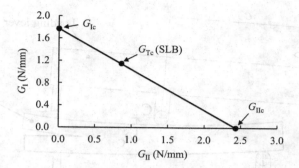

FIGURE 6.6 Plot of the linear energetic criterion defined from pure mode values (G_{Ic} and G_{IIc}) and the total fracture energy ensuing from the simulation of the SLB test.

validates the SLB as an adequate test for mixed-mode I+II fracture characterisation of cortical bone tissue.

6.2 NUMERICAL ANALYSIS OF THE MIXED-MODE BENDING (MMB) TEST

The SLB test is easy to perform, but it is characterised by a constant mode ratio leading to a sole point in the G_I–G_{II} space. To overcome this drawback, the eventual application of a miniaturised version of the mixed-mode bending (MMB) test will also be analysed. This test requires a complex apparatus, but it has the advantage of providing a wide range of mixed-mode ratios. The mode-mixity can be easily altered by changing the lever length of the loading apparatus (parameter c in Figure 6.7).

Additionally, the load applied to the specimen can be easily partitioned into mode I and mode II components. The MMB test can be viewed as a combination of the double cantilever beam (DCB) and ENF tests. The analysis of static equilibrium of the loading lever and of the specimen enables the partition of the MMB loading by a combination of mode I and II components used in those tests (Figure 6.8),

$$P_I = \left(\frac{3c - L}{4L}\right)P \text{ and } P_{II} = \left(\frac{c + L}{4L}\right)P \qquad (6.8)$$

The corresponding mode I and II displacements can also be obtained during the test [Oliveira et al, 2007]. The mode I displacement component (δ_I) is equal to the displacement at the specimen extremity (point E in Figure 6.7) and the mode II component is given by $\delta_{II} = \delta_C + \delta_I/4$, being C the loaded mid-span point of the specimen (Figure 6.7), and δ_C the displacement measured in that point.

The definition of the c value corresponding to a given mode ratio was performed by Reeder [2003] using the corrected beam theory proposed by Kinloch et al. [1993] to get the following relation:

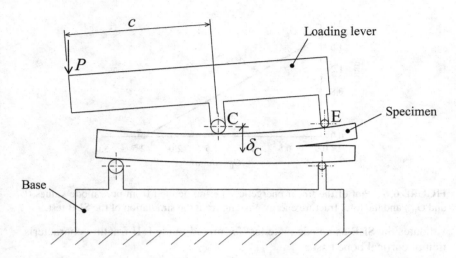

FIGURE 6.7 Schematic representation of the MMB test showing the lever length of the loading apparatus, c.

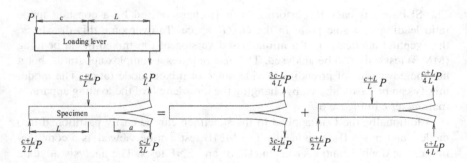

FIGURE 6.8 Loading partition (mode I and mode II) of the MMB test.

$$\frac{G_I}{G_{II}} = \frac{4}{3}\left(\frac{3c-L}{c+L}\right)^2\left(\frac{a+h\Delta}{a+0.42h\Delta}\right)^2 \qquad (6.9)$$

where Δ is a factor to account for root rotation effects given by [Kinloch et al., 1993]

$$\Delta = \sqrt{\frac{E_L}{11G_{LT}}\left[3-2\left(\frac{\Gamma}{1+\Gamma}\right)^2\right]} \quad \text{and} \quad \Gamma = 1.18\frac{\sqrt{E_L E_T}}{G_{LT}} \qquad (6.10)$$

with $2L$ standing for the useful specimen length a, for the current crack length and $2h$ for the specimen thickness.

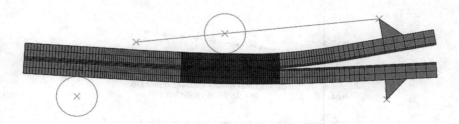

FIGURE 6.9   Finite element mesh used in the MMB test.

From Eq. (6.9), the value of c for a given mode ratio yields

$$c = \frac{L\left(1+\sqrt{F}\right)}{3-\sqrt{F}} \quad \text{with} \quad F = \frac{3}{4}\frac{\dfrac{G_I}{G_{II}}}{\left(\dfrac{a+h\Delta}{a+0.42h\Delta}\right)^2} \tag{6.11}$$

Numerical analyses employing a refined finite element mesh in the region of crack propagation (Figure 6.9) were accomplished considering three different mode ratios. The elastic properties, the fracture properties and the fracture criterion (Eq. 3.20 with $\gamma = 1$) were the ones used in the simulations of the SLB test. The values of loading components (P_I and P_{II}), corresponding displacements (δ_I and δ_{II}) and the crack length (a), were registered in the course of the numerical simulations for post-processing analysis. Three different mode-mixities were considered: predominant mode II ($G_{II}/G_T = 0.75$), equitable mode-mix ($G_{II}/G_T = 0.5$) and predominant mode I loading ($G_{II}/G_T = 0.25$).

Figure 6.10 plots the evolution of the mode I and mode II compliances (C_I and C_{II}) versus crack length (a), considering the case of predominant mode II that is achieved imposing the distance $c = 17.31$ mm (Figure 6.8) obtained from Eq. (6.11). These relationships were approximated with third-degree polynomials, thus enabling differentiation relative to crack length to be used in the Irwin–Kies equation (Eq. 3.5). The evolution of the strain energy release rate components is plotted in Figure 6.11a and the mode-mixity as a function of the crack length in Figure 6.11b. A plateau trend is observed in all cases, meaning that self-similar crack growth conditions are fulfilled for a given crack extent.

A similar procedure was followed considering $c = 24.63$ mm and $c = 44.59$ mm giving rise to $G_{II}/G_T = 0.5$ and $G_{II}/G_T = 0.25$, respectively. Although slight variations on the values of G_I and G_{II} as a function of crack length are observed due to polynomial fitting inaccuracies, it should be emphasised that the mode-mixity G_{II}/G_T is almost constant and well captured in both cases (Figures 6.12 and 6.13). These results lead to the conclusion that the MMB test is a valid option for fracture characterisation of cortical bone under mixed-mode I+II loading.

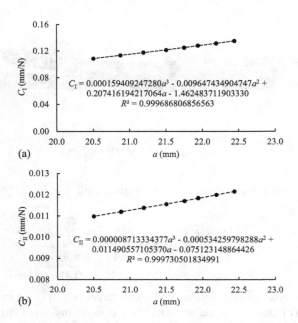

FIGURE 6.10 Evolution of compliances (C_I and C_II) as a function of crack length considering $c = 17.31$ mm.

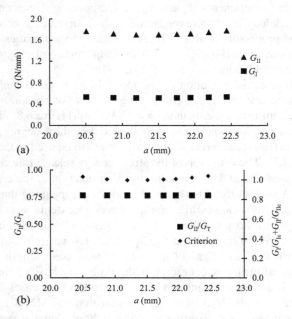

FIGURE 6.11 Evolution as a function of crack length of (a) strain energy release rate components (G_I and G_II) and (b) mode-mixity ($G_\mathrm{II}/G_\mathrm{T}$) and fracture criterion considering $c = 17.31$ mm.

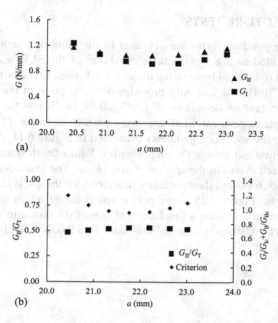

FIGURE 6.12 Evolution as a function of crack length of (a) strain energy release rate components (G_I and G_{II}) and (b) mode-mixity (G_{II}/G_T) and fracture criterion considering $c = 24.63$ mm.

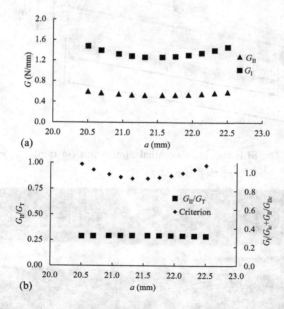

FIGURE 6.13 Evolution as a function of crack length of (a) strain energy release rate components (G_I and G_{II}) and (b) mode-mixity (G_{II}/G_T) and fracture criterion considering $c = 44.59$ mm.

6.3 SLB FRACTURE TESTS

Considering the good performance obtained in the numerical analysis (Section 6.1), it was decided to use a miniaturised version of the SLB test for fracture characterisation of cortical bone tissue under mixed-mode I+II loading conditions [Pereira et al., 2014]. The test only provides one sole point in the G_I–G_{II} space leading to a constant mode-mixity of $G_{II}/G_T \approx 0.43$, but it has the advantage of being very simple to perform. SLB tests were performed in the TL fracture system considering the specimen geometry presented in Figure 6.14. As in previous cases, two longitudinal groves (V-shape) with 0.5 mm depth were machined to induce some crack extent in the specimen mid-plane. The execution of the notch and the pre-crack followed the procedure described for the DCB test.

The SLB tests (Figure 6.15) were performed considering an acquisition frequency of 5 Hz and imposing a displacement rate of 0.1 mm/min using a servo-electrical material testing system (MicroTester INSTRON® 5848) with a 2 kN load cell.

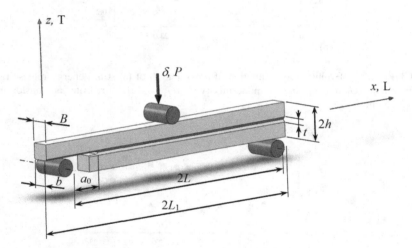

FIGURE 6.14 The SLB specimen nominal dimensions (in mm): $2L_1 = 65$; $2L = 60$, $2h = 6$; $t = 1$; $B = 3.3$; $b = 2.3$; $a_0 = 18$.

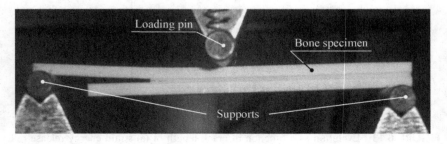

FIGURE 6.15 The SLB testing setup.

Figure 6.16 reveals details of the fractured region. Detail A shows the existence of opening and shear relative displacements evidencing that mixed-mode I+II loading is present. Detail B highlights the difficulty of crack tip identification making dubious the evaluation of its length that is necessary to determine the fracture energy components in classical data reduction methods.

The fracture surfaces of a tested SLB bone specimen were observed by scanning electron microscopy (Philips-FEI Quanta 400). Three regions can be observed (Figure 6.17). Region A corresponds to the pre-crack surface initiated by a saw and adjusted by a sharp blade and Region C identifies the lateral longitudinal grooves. Region B is the fracture surface under mixed-mode I+II loading, which can be viewed in more detail in Figure 6.18.

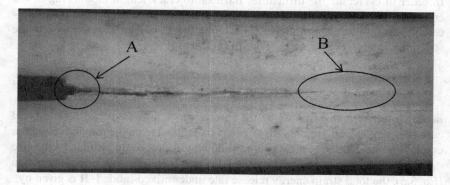

FIGURE 6.16 Crack details revealing opening and shear displacements at the notch tip (A) and undefined crack tip position (B).

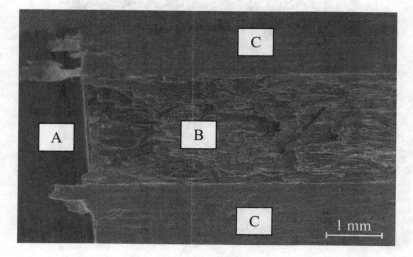

FIGURE 6.17 Fracture surface of the SLB test: A – initial pre-crack; B – mixed-mode I+II fracture surface; C – lateral grooves.

It can be observed that the fracture surface is rough and irregular in general, which is explained by the internal bone microstructure. Detail A of Figure 6.18 shows the combination of peel (mode I) and shear (mode II) effects induced by the mixed-mode I+II loading. The peel loading induces a lifting effect and the shear loading gives rise to a preferential longitudinal alignment of the fractured microstructures. The combination of these two effects is visible in detail A of Figure 6.18, where an inclined fractured microstructure can be identified.

6.3.1 COMPLIANCE-BASED BEAM METHOD (CBBM) APPLIED TO THE SLB TEST

In order to overcome the difficulties intrinsic to crack length monitoring in the course of the test (detail B in Figure 6.16), an equivalent crack length-based procedure was developed for the SLB test. Using the Timoshenko beam theory, the specimen compliance becomes [Pereira et al., 2014],

$$C = \frac{7a^3 + 2L^3}{8E_L Bh^3} + \frac{3(a+2L)}{20G_{LT}Bh} \tag{6.12}$$

in which the E_L is determined by the inverse procedure described for the DCB case. The equivalent crack length (a_e) can be obtained from the previous equation employing the Matlab® software and following a procedure similar to the one described in Section 4.4.1. By combining Eq. (6.12) with the Irwin–Kies equation (Eq. 3.5), the total strain energy release rate under mixed-mode I+II is given by

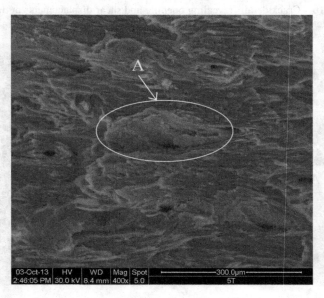

FIGURE 6.18 Microphotography of the fracture surface; detail A highlights shear and peel effects.

$$G_{\mathrm{T}} = \frac{21P^2 a_{\mathrm{e}}^2}{16E_{\mathrm{L}}Bbh^3} + \frac{3P^2}{40G_{\mathrm{LT}}Bbh} \tag{6.13}$$

The mode I and mode II components can be obtained by a partition method proposed in de Moura et al. [2017], which leads to

$$G_{\mathrm{I}} = \frac{12P^2 a_{\mathrm{e}}^2}{16E_{\mathrm{L}}Bbh^3} + \frac{3P^2}{40G_{\mathrm{LT}}Bbh} \quad ; \quad G_{\mathrm{II}} = \frac{9P^2 a_{\mathrm{e}}^2}{16E_{\mathrm{L}}Bbh^3} \tag{6.14}$$

This procedure avoids cumbersome and inaccurate crack length monitoring and permits to account indirectly for the influence of a non-negligible fracture process zone.

Figure 6.19 presents the ensemble of load–displacement curves of the eight valid tests. A large scatter is visible that is normal in a natural material like bone characterised by anisotropy and internal heterogeneity.

The CBBM was applied to load–displacement data in order to obtain the corresponding R-curves, i.e., $G_{\mathrm{I}} = f(a_{\mathrm{e}})$ and $G_{\mathrm{II}} = f(a_{\mathrm{e}})$ given by Eqs. (6.14), considering the equivalent crack length obtained by means of Eq. (6.12). Owing to the observed scatter, it was decided to plot the average smoothed experimental R-curves with the respective standard deviation throughout the curves (Figure 6.20).

The energy release rate tends to a plateau, representative of self-similar crack propagation. Under such circumstances, the crack grows naturally with the fully developed fracture process zone ahead of its tip, which is crucial for a correct evaluation of the total fracture energy, as well as its mode I and II components. Table 6.1 summarises the results of the eight valid tests. A scatter of around 15% was obtained, which is good in the context of a natural material as is the case of bone. The global mode-mixity using the average energy components (Table 6.1) is $G_{\mathrm{II}}/G_{\mathrm{T}} = 0.425$, which is in agreement with the value expected for the SLB test.

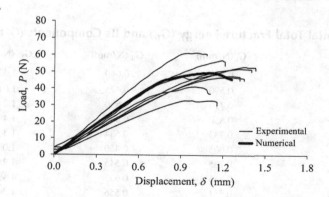

FIGURE 6.19 Experimental and numerical load–displacement curves of the SLB tests in bovine cortical bone.

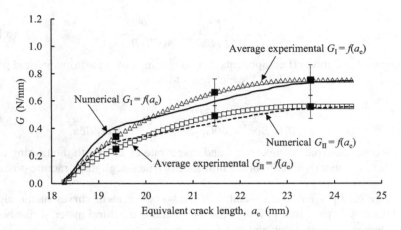

FIGURE 6.20 Experimental averaged and numerical R-curves of the SLB test applied to mixed-mode I+II fracture characterisation of bovine cortical bone.

The average values of fracture energy in pure modes (G_{Ic} = 1.77 N/mm) determined by Morais et al. [2010] and G_{IIc} = 2.25 N/mm obtained by Dourado et al. [2013] and the average fracture energy components presented in Table 6.1 were used to determine the fracture envelope representative of this set of bovine cortical bone specimens. In order to take into account the material scatter, Figure 6.21 plots the fracture envelopes considering three power laws (Eq. 3.20) with different exponents: γ = 0.62 (dashed line in Figure 6.21) describes the average trend, while the other ones, γ = 0.52 and γ = 0.72 (solid lines in Figure 6.21), bound the extreme values of fracture energy under mixed-mode I+II loading obtained with the SLB test.

TABLE 6.1

Experimental Total Fracture Energy (G_{Tc}) and Its Components (G_I and G_{II})

Specimen	G_I (N/mm)	G_{II} (N/mm)	G_{Tc} (N/mm)
1	0.880	0.640	1.520
2	0.590	0.425	1.015
3	0.710	0.530	1.240
4	0.850	0.640	1.490
5	0.783	0.584	1.367
6	0.605	0.450	1.055
7	0.735	0.545	1.280
8	0.855	0.635	1.490
Average	0.751	0.556	1.307
CoV (%)	14.9	15.3	15.02

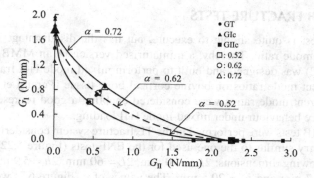

FIGURE 6.21 Fracture envelopes in the G_I–G_{II} space obtained for bovine cortical bone.

With the objective of confirming the validity of the followed procedure, a finite element analysis was performed. A refined mesh containing 944 eight-node plane stress solid elements (width B) and 108 six-node cohesive elements (different width b to account for the lateral grooves, according to Figure 6.14 was used. A version of the mixed-mode I+II cohesive zone model presented in Chapter 3 (Figure 3.4) based on previous works (Table 6.2) was considered. These works have shown that for cortical bone tissue a bilinear softening law is appropriate for mode I, while a trapezoidal law is better suited for mode II loading.

The load–displacement numerical curve considering $\gamma = 0.62$ is included in Figure 6.19. It can be verified that the numerical curve represents well the experimental trend. The corresponding R-curves were obtained by the proposed CBBM and included in Figure 6.20. An excellent agreement between the numerical and experimental averaged curves can be observed, especially in the plateau regions of the fracture energy components, reflecting self-similar crack growth.

The numerical values referring to the three power laws ($\gamma = 0.52$, 0.62 and 0.72) were included in Figure 6.21 (unfilled marks). Each numerical result agrees with the corresponding fracture envelope enabling the validation of the proposed procedure. Actually, this agreement reflects that the proposed data reduction method and miniaturised version of the SLB test enable to reproduce accurately the used power law.

TABLE 6.2
Cohesive Parameters of the Pure Mode (I and II) Laws for Bovine Cortical Bone [Morais et al., 2010; Pereira et al., 2011; Dourado et al., 2013]

	$\sigma_{1,i}$ (MPa)	$\delta_{2,i}$ (mm)	$\delta_{3,i}$ (mm)	$\sigma_{3,i}$ (MPa)	G_{ic} (N/mm)
Mode I ($i = $ I)	36	36E-6	0.07	4.9	1.77
Mode II ($i = $ II)	59.5	0.018	0.04	26.5	2.25

6.4 MMB FRACTURE TESTS

The SLB test is quite simple to execute, but has the disadvantage of providing a fixed mode ratio. Thereby, a miniaturised version of an MMB apparatus (Figure 6.22) was designed and built to perform mixed-mode I+II fracture tests with different mode ratios on bovine cortical bone tissue [Pereira et al., 2016]. Three different mode ratios were considered enabling a good representation of bone fracture behaviour under mixed-mode I+II loading.

The MMB tests were performed in the TL fracture system considering a specimen geometry similar to the one used for the ENF tests (Figure 5.22) considering the following dimensions: $2L_1 = 70$ mm, $2L = 60$ mm, $2h = 5.9$ mm, $b = 1.6$ mm, $B = 2.7$ mm and $a_0 = 20.5$ mm. The values of c (Figure 6.7) were chosen according to Eqs (6.11) in order to propitiate predominant mode II loading (15 specimens with $c = 18$ mm leading to $G_{II}/G_T = 0.72$), equitable loading modes (17 specimens with $c = 29$ mm giving rise to $G_{II}/G_T = 0.41$) and predominant mode I

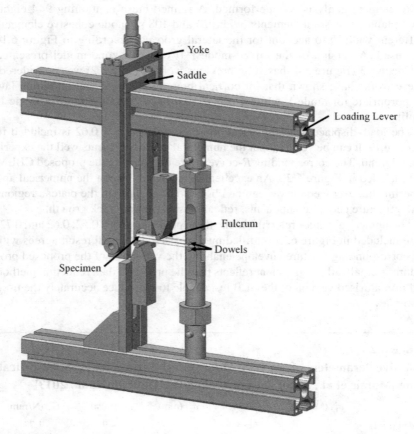

FIGURE 6.22 Schematic representation of the miniaturised version of the MMB text apparatus built for cortical bone fracture characterisation under mixed-mode I+II loading.

(10 specimens with $c = 44$ mm corresponding to $G_{II}/G_T = 0.25$). The MMB fracture tests (Figure 6.23) were performed using a servo-electrical material testing system (MicroTester INSTRON® 5848) with a constant displacement rate of 0.5 mm/min. A 2 kN load cell was used and the data acquisition frequency was set equal to 5 Hz.

6.4.1 COMPLIANCE-BASED BEAM METHOD (CBBM) APPLIED TO THE MMB TEST

The data reduction method used in Section 6.2 requires crack length monitoring in the course of the test in order to establish the compliance calibration (Figure 6.10). Although the current crack length is easily accessible in a finite element analysis, as done in Section 6.2, the same does not happen during experimental tests. An alternative to solve this difficulty is to implement the equivalent crack length procedure described for DCB and ENF tests (Figure 6.8). In fact, the equations obtained for DCB and ENF tests using Timoshenko beam theory can be used to obtain the equations for MMB tests taking into account the partition modes procedure (Figure 6.8). In this context, Eqs (4.4) and (5.5) can be employed to establish the $C_I = \delta_I/P_I = f(a)$ and $C_{II} = \delta_{II}/P_{II} = f(a)$ relationships, respectively. It should be noted that P_I, P_{II} are obtained by Eqs (6.8) and δ_I, δ_{II} require the measurement of the displacements at specimen extremity and at its mid-span (points E and C in Figure 6.7, respectively) in the course of the MMB test. The R-curves of the mode I and II components of the fracture energy are obtained following the procedure described for the DCB and ENF tests in Sections 4.4.1 and 5.6.1, respectively (Eqs (4.10) and (5.7)). This procedure avoids the undesirable and inaccurate task of crack length monitoring during the test, which is achieved with Eqs. (4.4–4.8) for the DCB test, and Eq. (5.6) for the ENF test.

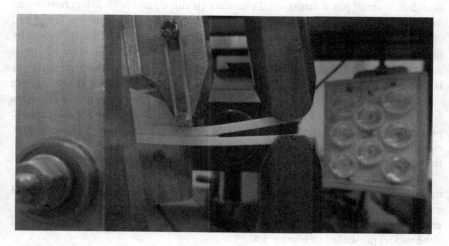

FIGURE 6.23 MMB test applied to bovine cortical bone tissue.

Figure 6.24a–c plots the load–displacement curves of the three mode-mixi-ties analysed, and Figure 6.24d shows a typical curve for each case allowing a clear visualisation of the differences between each test group. The corresponding R-curves for each mode component are obtained (Figure 6.25) applying the CBBM. In all cases, a steady-state plateau region can be identified meaning that stable crack growth has occurred for a given crack extent. Consistent results were obtained for the two former cases (Figures 6.24a, b and 6.25a–d), but a larger scatter is visible for the mode I predominant case (Figures 6.24c and 6.25e, f). The higher instability of this test probably explains such behaviour.

Tables 6.3–6.5 list all the values of valid MMB tests. Small differences were observed among the predicted mode-mixities and the ones really obtained, which is a good result for a natural material like bone. The coefficient of variation of fracture energy components is acceptable for the two former cases (Tables 6.3 and 6.4). However, the scatter for the $G_{II}/G_T = 0.25$ case was higher (Table 6.5), namely on the mode II strain energy release rate component, owing to difficulties associated with pronounced instability at crack starting advance.

The fracture envelope obtained for this set of bovine cortical bone, tested with the MMB, is plotted in Figure 6.26. Squared marks identify the average value of fracture energy for each mode ratio. For a better consistency of results, DCB and ENF fracture tests were also performed to determine the pure mode fracture energies in mode I and II, respectively, of this set of bovine femurs, and the average values were included in the plot. Despite the relevant scatter observed, it can be concluded that the linear energetic criterion (exponent $\gamma = 1.0$ in Eq. 3.20) is a good approach for $G_{II}/G_T = 0.25$ and $G_{II}/G_T = 0.72$ cases, being somewhat conservative for $G_{II}/G_T = 0.41$. Consequently, this criterion was adopted in the finite element analysis performed for validation of the followed procedure.

A two-dimensional finite element analysis including cohesive zone modelling was performed aiming to validate the followed procedure. A mesh of 2426 two-dimensional plane stress solid elements (width B) and with 218 cohesive elements (width b) was employed (Figure 6.9). The loading apparatus was simulated considering cylindrical rigid bodies and a loading beam tied to the specimen by means of a triangular rigid body (Figure 6.9). Contact surfaces were assumed between the cylindrical rigid bodies and the specimen to prevent interpenetration. Boundary conditions consist of clamping the bottom supports and imposing a vertical displacement to the beam's right extremity. Specimen average dimensions were considered for each mode-mixity set of tests. Table 6.6 lists the used elastic properties. The longitudinal elastic modulus (E_L) was adjusted by an inverse procedure for each mode-mixity series of tests, to reproduce the elastic stiffness and the remaining elastic properties were taken from Morais et al. [2010].

Table 6.7 presents the cohesive parameters used in this analysis. The pure modes cohesive laws were determined by an inverse procedure applied to DCB and ENF tests. For simplicity, two bilinear softening relationships were considered, meaning that point 2 coincides with point 1 in the cohesive mixed-mode I+II zone model presented in Figure 3.4.

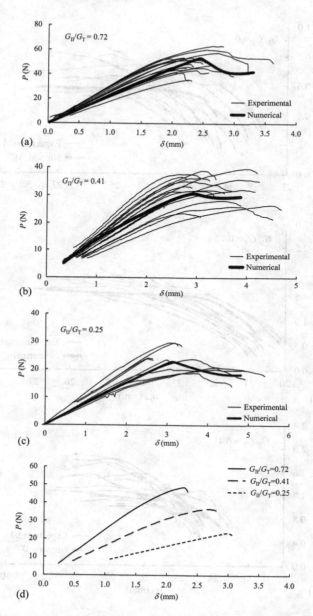

FIGURE 6.24 Load–displacement curves of the MMB test for the mode ratios analysed: (a) G_{II}/G_T=0.72, (b) G_{II}/G_T=0.41, (c) G_{II}/G_T=0.25 and (d) typical curve for each case.

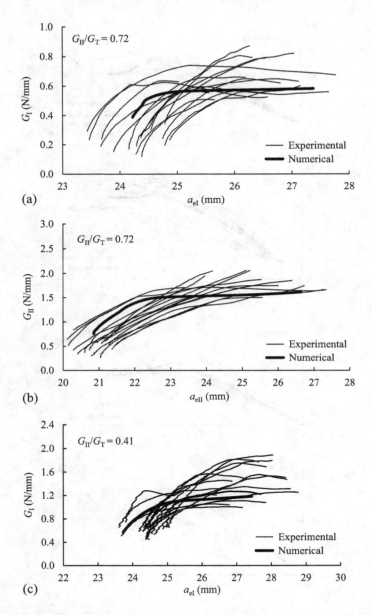

FIGURE 6.25 *R*-curves of the two mode components of fracture energy for the three mode ratios analysed (0.72, 0.41 and 0.25) showing: (a, c, e) G_I *vs* a_{eI}, (b, d, f) G_{II} *vs* a_{eII}.

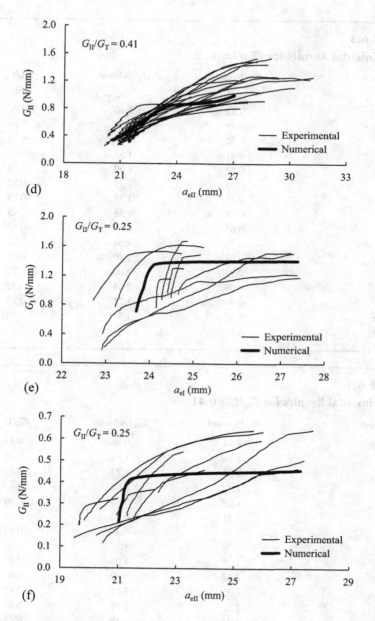

(d)

(e)

(f)

FIGURE 6.25 (Continued)

TABLE 6.3
Experimental Results for $G_{II}/G_T=0.72$

Specimen	G_I (N/mm)	G_{II} (N/mm)	G_{II}/G_T
1	0.83	1.92	0.70
2	0.72	2.10	0.74
3	0.59	2.10	0.78
4	0.52	1.37	0.72
5	0.61	1.53	0.72
6	0.57	1.50	0.73
7	0.65	1.71	0.72
8	0.62	1.85	0.75
9	0.57	1.56	0.73
10	0.63	1.66	0.72
11	0.79	2.04	0.72
12	0.51	1.30	0.72
13	0.79	2.00	0.72
14	0.78	2.05	0.72
15	0.65	1.71	0.73
Average	0.67	1.77	0.73
CoV (%)	15.6	15.2	2.6

TABLE 6.4
Experimental Results for $G_{II}/G_T=0.41$

Specimen	G_I (N/mm)	G_{II} (N/mm)	G_{II}/G_T
1	1.14	0.86	0.43
2	1.26	1.05	0.45
3	1.54	1.27	0.45
4	1.4	0.95	0.40
5	1.05	0.88	0.46
6	1.21	0.92	0.43
7	1.27	0.85	0.40
8	1.78	1.5	0.46
9	1.25	1.08	0.46
10	1.12	0.89	0.44
11	1.53	1.09	0.42
12	1.32	1.19	0.47
13	1.44	1.18	0.45
14	1.82	1.37	0.43
15	1.74	1.36	0.44
16	1.53	1.16	0.43
17	1.04	0.78	0.43
Average	1.45	1.14	0.44
CoV (%)	17.0	18.5	4.6

TABLE 6.5

Experimental Results for $G_{II}/G_T=0.25$

Specimen	G_I (N/mm)	G_{II} (N/mm)	G_{II}/G_T
1	1.46	0.39	0.21
2	1.3	0.34	0.21
3	1.13	0.29	0.20
4	1.66	0.52	0.24
5	1.6	0.61	0.28
6	1.14	0.44	0.28
7	1.45	0.62	0.30
8	1.18	0.45	0.28
9	1.51	0.62	0.29
10	1.42	0.58	0.29
Average	1.385	0.486	0.26
CoV (%)	13.7	25.1	14.8

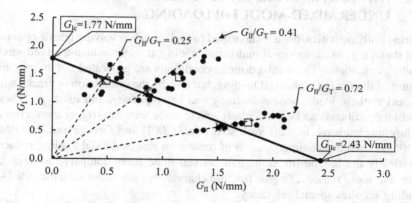

FIGURE 6.26 Fracture envelope of bovine cortical bone obtained using the MMB test (squared marks identify the average values for each mode ratio and diagonal crosses the numerical values).

These laws were used in the numerical model along with the value of the exponent ($\gamma = 1.0$) determined by the fracture envelope (Figure 6.26). The numerical load–displacement curves and the corresponding R-curves were included in Figures 6.24 and 6.25. In general, it can be stated that these numerical curves represent well the observed experimental trends. The numerical values of fracture energy (identified by crosses) were also included in Figure 6.26. It can be observed that they are close to the linear energetic criterion ($\gamma = 1.0$). This statement validates the procedure and the MMB test in the context of mixed-mode I+II fracture characterisation of cortical bone tissue.

TABLE 6.6
Elastic Properties of Cortical Bone Tissue

E_L (MPa)	E_T (MPa)	G_{LT} (MPa)	ν_{LT}
12,000–13,500	9,550	4,740	0.37

TABLE 6.7
Parameters of the Cohesive Laws for Mode I and Mode II

	$\sigma_{i,1}$ (MPa)	$\delta_{i,3}$ (mm)	$\sigma_{i,3}$ (MPa)	G_{ic} (N/mm)
Mode I (i = I)	47.3	0.05	9.99	1.77
Mode II (i = II)	58.0	0.05	22.16	2.43

6.5 FATIGUE/FRACTURE CHARACTERISATION TESTS UNDER MIXED-MODE I+II LOADING

During daily activities, bone is submitted to cyclic loads involving tensile opening and shear, e.g., axial–torsional multiaxial loading, thereby inducing mixed-mode loading conditions. These mixed-mode conditions are generated not only by the nature of the *in vivo* multiaxial loading, but also by the orientation of cracks with respect to these loads, bone anisotropy and heterogeneity, and its shape. These loading conditions can be particularly severe since they can trigger more critical failure mechanisms. In fact, Vashishth et al. [2001] and George and Vashishth [2006] observed that superposition of torsion on reversed axial loading reduces drastically the fatigue life of human cortical bone when compared to uniaxial tests. For these reasons, fatigue/fracture characterisation under mixed-mode I+II loading acquires special relevancy.

The objective of the following fatigue/fracture tests is to identify a suitable fatigue crack propagation law, as a function of the mode-mixity, to predict bone fatigue life. In particular, the modified Paris law will be applied and the respective coefficients will be identified as a function of mixed-mode ratio.

6.5.1 SLB FATIGUE TESTS ON BOVINE CORTICAL BONE TISSUE

The MMB test allows a wide variation of the mode-mixity, but it requires a complex apparatus that can originate some problems under high-cycle fatigue loading. Therefore, the SLB test was chosen to perform fatigue/fracture characterisation under mixed-mode I+II loading of bovine cortical bone tissue taking into account its simplicity.

Fifteen SLB specimens were carefully prepared following the procedure previously described. Preliminary quasi-static SLB tests were performed (Figure 6.27)

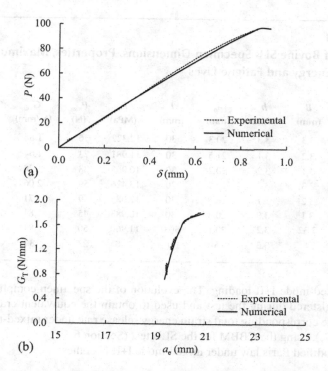

FIGURE 6.27 Results of an SLB test on bovine bone: (a) load–displacement curves and (b) *R*-curves.

under displacement control with a rate of 0.075 mm/min until a quite small crack growth is achieved, which occurs close to maximum load (P_u). Specimens with longitudinal grooves and with hydration were considered and the corresponding load–displacement curves were registered. This strategy allowed estimating the value of $P_{max} = 0.5P_u$ to be applied in the fatigue/fracture tests and the total fracture energy under mixed-mode I+II loading (G_{Tc}), employing the described CBBM.

The average values of G_{Ic}, G_{IIc} and G_{Tc} ensuing from the quasi-static DCB (Table 4.3), ENF (Table 5.4) and SLB tests (Table 6.8), respectively, were plotted in Figure 6.28. It can be observed that the power law energetic criterion with exponent $\gamma = 1.0$ (linear energetic criterion) reproduces well the fracture envelope for this set of bone samples and it was used as input in the numerical simulations to define the fracture energy (G_{Tc}) for the mixed-mode occurring at each integration point.

Fatigue/fracture SLB tests were performed after the quasi-static tests under loading control, $P_{max} = P_u/2$, load ratio $R = P_{min}/P_{max} = 0.1$ and a frequency of 2 Hz. Continuous irrigation was ensured during the tests. Despite this fact, some specimens failed by premature arm rupture or crack deviation from their initial plane, but six valid results were obtained to evaluate the fatigue/fracture behaviour

TABLE 6.8

Resume of Bovine SLB Specimen Dimensions, Properties, Maximum Load, Fracture Energy and Fatigue Lives

Specimen	B (mm)	h (mm)	a_0 (mm)	L (mm)	E_L (MPa)	P_{max} (N)	G_{Tc} (N/mm)	Fatigue life (Cycles)
1	3.3	3.3	20.3	30	12,322	36	1.88	59,822
2	3.2	3.1	21.5	30	11,981	73	1.64	44,735
3	3.1	3.2	20.2	30	10,963	38	1.78	48,507
4	3.3	3.2	19.7	30	13,426	59	2.06	50,982
5	3.2	3.1	18.5	30	12,085	49	1.71	47,946
6	3.1	3.0	20.3	30	10,983	45	1.81	45,820
Average	3.32	3.2	20.1	30.0	11,960	50	1.81	49,635
CoV (%)	4	3.3	5	0	8	28	8	11

under mixed-mode I+II loading. The evolution of the specimen compliance $C = f(N)$ is registered during the test and used to obtain the equivalent crack length (a_e) and the corresponding total strain energy release rate under mixed-mode I+II loading (G_T), using the CBBM for the SLB test (Section 6.3.1).

The modified Paris law under mixed-mode I+II becomes

$$\frac{dA_e}{dN} = C_{1,m}\left(\frac{\Delta G_T}{G_{Tc}}\right)^{C_{2,m}} = C_{1,m}\left(\frac{G_{T,max}(1-R)^2}{G_{Tc}}\right)^{C_{2,m}} \quad (6.15)$$

where ΔG_T and $G_{T,max}$ are the variation and maximum values of the mixed-mode I+II strain energy release rate in a cycle, respectively, G_{Tc} is the mixed-mode I+II

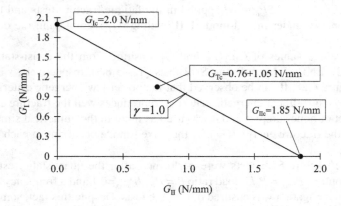

FIGURE 6.28 Fracture envelope obtained from the average values G_{Ic}, G_{IIc} and G_{Tc} of bovine cortical bone tissue.

fracture energy for a given mode-mixity and $C_{1,m}$, $C_{2,m}$ are the Paris law coefficients under mixed-mode I+II loading.

Figure 6.29 shows an SLB specimen after testing, revealing the existence of some crack extent at the specimen mid-plane, which is crucial for a truthful evaluation of fracture toughness under mixed-mode I+II loading.

The CBBM of the SLB test (Section 6.3.1) was applied to the $C = f(N)$ curve (Figure 6.30a) to obtain the evolution of the equivalent crack length (Figure 6.30b) and of the total strain energy release rate (Figure 6.30c), both as a function of the number of cycles. The profiles of the curves are similar to each other and depict a smooth increase of fatigue damage up to 50,000 cycles, approximately, followed by an abrupt failure. The corresponding evolution of the damaged area growth rate (dA_c/dN – mm²/cycle) as a function of energy ratio ($\Delta G_T/G_{Tc}$) for the region of stable crack growth is presented in Figure 6.30d in a bi-logarithmic scale. A monotonic rising trend is obtained representing cumulative damage effects as a function of time.

The evolution of compliance normalised by the specimen dimensions with the number of cycles is gathered in Figure 6.31a. The normalisation is based on the compliance equation (Eq. 6.12) and aims to reduce the influence of specimen dimensions on the scatter observed on its initial compliance. Despite this strategy, some scatter is observed on initial normalised compliance and on the predicted fatigue lives. The adjustment of a power law to all valid results (Figure 6.31b) enables defining the coefficients of the modified Paris law ($C_{1m} = 0.499$ mm²/cycle and $C_{2m} = 7.215$) for fatigue/fracture behaviour of this set of bovine bone specimens under mixed-mode I+II loading. Table 6.8 summarises specimen dimensions, properties, maximum load, fracture energy and fatigue lives of the valid test results.

Figure 6.32 presents the values of the Paris law coefficients obtained in the three fatigue/fracture tests (DCB, ENF and SLB). Two functions were considered

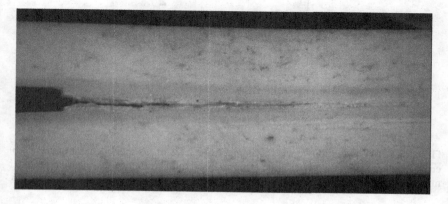

FIGURE 6.29 SLB specimen after testing revealing some crack extend (Δa) under self-similar conditions.

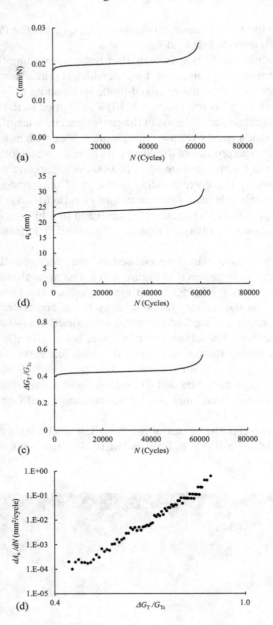

FIGURE 6.30 Evolution versus the number of cycles of (a) specimen compliance; (b) equivalent crack length; (c) variation of normalised total strain energy release rate under mixed-mode I+II loading; and (d) damaged area growth rate as a function of energy ratio.

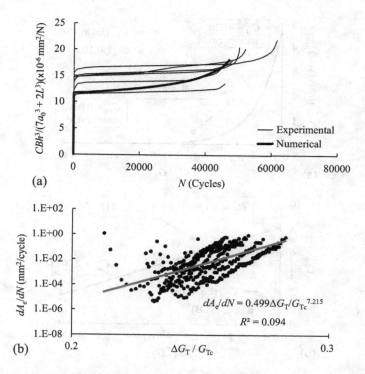

(a)

(b)

FIGURE 6.31 (a) Normalised compliance versus number of cycles for the valid tests on bovine bone and (b) fatigue damage growth (dA_e/dN – mm²/cycle) as a function of $\Delta G_T/G_{Tc}$ in a bi-logarithmic representation.

in order to describe, approximately, the variation of those coefficients as a function of the mode-mixity (G_{II}/G_T),

$$\ln(C_{1m}) = \ln(C_{1I}) + \frac{\left[\ln(C_{1II}) - \ln(C_{1I})\right]G_{II}}{G_T}$$

$$C_{2m} = C_{2I} + \frac{(C_{2II} - C_{2I})G_{II}}{G_T}$$

(6.16)

These relations establish a linear evolution for the coefficient C_{2m} and a linear evolution in a logarithmic scale for C_{1m}, and they were utilised in the numerical model to deal with mixed-mode variation at the integration points during loading.

A numerical analysis was performed for the SLB fatigue tests considering the modified Paris law for mixed-mode I+II loading (Eq. 6.16). The critical fracture energy (G_{Tc}) for any mode-mixity (α) is defined by Eq. (3.22) considering $\gamma = 1.0$ (Figure 6.26). The parameters of the Paris law ($C_{1,m}$ and $C_{2,m}$) for the mode-mixity (G_{II}/G_T) existing at the actual integration point are defined as a function of the

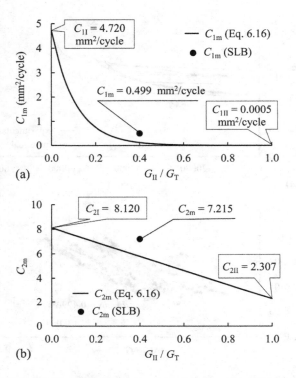

FIGURE 6.32 Plot of C_{1m} and C_{2m} as a function of the mode-mixity (Eq. 6.16), and the Paris law parameters ensuing from the SLB test for bovine bone (Figure 6.31b).

corresponding pure mode values ($C_{1,i}$ and $C_{2,i}$ with i = I, II) and are given by Eqs. (6.16). It should be noted that the local mode-mixities at the integration points change in the course of the test and from point to point [de Moura et al., 2016], which reinforces the relevance of the relations depicted in Eqs. (6.16). The numerical curve showing the normalised compliance versus the number of cycles was included in Figure 6.31a. It can be stated that it represents well the experimental trends, pointing to a fatigue life around 50,000 cycles, which is in close agreement with the average experimental value (Table 6.8). This shows the suitability of the numerical model and of the employed procedure to deal with mixed-mode I+II fatigue/fracture characterisation of cortical bone tissue. In fact, it can be stated that the numerical model reproduces well the experimental trends, which makes it a suitable tool to deal with studies involving fatigue/fracture characterisation under mixed-mode I+II loading of cortical bone tissue.

6.6 SUMMARY

This chapter covers the mixed-mode I+II quasi-static and fatigue/fracture characterisation of cortical bone tissue. An initial analysis of the mixed-mode I+II fracture tests used in the context of cortical bone tissue revealed that they suffer from several shortcomings in terms of adequately characterising the mixed-mode

I+II fracture of bone. In contrast, numerical analyses on the single-leg bending and mixed-mode bending fracture tests revealed that they are suitable for mixed-mode I+II fracture studies on this material. Both tests were used experimentally in order to define the fracture envelope under mixed-mode I+II quasi-static loading. Appropriate data reduction methods based on the equivalent crack length concept were developed to simplify the experimental determination of the strain energy release rate. Fatigue/fracture analyses were carried out using the single-leg bending tests due to their simplicity. The coefficients of the modified Paris law for mixed-mode I+II loading and the fatigue lives were obtained. Two functions correlating the Paris law coefficients in the pure (I and II) and mixed-mode I+II loading were adopted aiming to describe, approximately, the variation of those coefficients as a function of the mode ratio. These functions were used as input in the numerical model to deal with mixed-mode variation at the integration points during simulation. It was concluded that the predicted fatigue life is in agreement with the experimental trends.

7 Practical Applications

As discussed in Sections 1.3 and 3, bone fracture is one of the most important health problems in today's society. Several different types of fractures, e.g., transverse, spiral, oblique, compression, greenstick, comminuted and segmental ones, may result from daily activities and trauma, when bone mechanical strength is exceeded due to applied loading [Sheng et al., 2019]. Osteosynthesis metal plates and bicortical screws, in contact with the wall of long bones, are frequently used to promote bone regeneration, while offering the required mechanical stabilisation and fracture alignment. Therefore, it is necessary to consider bone immobilisation based on mechanical fixation systems that employ wires, screws, grids and/or plates, which are put in contact with the periosteum [Zhou et al., 2017]. These internal fixation systems should be able to respond adequately to temporary injuries preserving the complex tissue organisation (e.g., vascularity). Consequently, for all of these reasons, it becomes relevant to optimise the fixation setup either functionally and geometrically. Osteosynthesis metal plates and bicortical screws, in contact with the wall of long bones, are frequently used to promote bone regeneration, contributing to mechanical stabilisation and fracture alignment. In clinical practice, the screws are used to perform the direct fixation of bone segments or to assure the fixation of internal or external plates, necessary for the immobilisation of bone fractures. The placement of screws during the fixation of bone pieces should be done, whenever possible, in the centre of the bone, since this allows for a more secure retention of those pieces. The arrangement of bicortical screws can induce important stress concentrations in the screw–bone interface, making crucial the evaluation of damage parameters in this region. In fact, it has been found that this interface has a considerable impact on the local stress–strain fields near the screws, leading to different mechanical responses of bone damage and ultimately screw loosening [MacLeod et al., 2012].

The objective of this chapter is to describe some applications of the methodologies exposed in previous chapters regarding immobilisation of bone fractures. In fact, finite element analysis including cohesive zone modelling can be used as predictive tools in the simulation of the structural behaviour of the bone fixation setups employed for the immobilisation systems used to treat bone fractures. The objective is to identify the critical regions and perform a progressive damage analysis allowing the detection of the riskiest zones.

Three different types of fractures will be analysed in this chapter: transverse, oblique and comminuted. All these fractures were immobilised by dynamic compression plates (DCPs) fastened to the cortical bone tissue using surgical screws.

   DOI: 10.1201/9781003375081-7

7.1 TRANSVERSE FRACTURE

7.1.1 EXPERIMENTAL TESTS

Transverse fracture is one of the most common types of bone fractures. It is characterised by a fracture plane perpendicular to the longitudinal bone axis (Figure 7.1) and is considered one of the most simple to immobilise.

In the present case, the right femur of an adult goat was used for the study. The procedures inherent to specimens' preparation were similar to the ones described previously for fracture tests. The fracture line was simulated by an osteotomy using a bone cutter saw.

One of the techniques used in Orthopaedics, in the stabilisation and repair of bone fractures, consists of using DCPs with the purpose of promoting a stable connection between bone segments that are separated (Figure 7.2). These fixation plates are made of stainless steel or titanium, with standardised characteristic dimensions, regarding thickness, width and length, as well as the alignment of the holes for the application of cortical screws, usually made of the same material.

The DCPs originally had a flat configuration, but it was plastically deformed, using pliers suitable for Orthopaedics practice. This procedure was performed before tightening the screws, in order to increase the contact surface with the bone, therefore promoting the alignment of the bone pieces and allowing for the best possible vascularisation of the damaged area. Subsequently, eight bicortical screws (diameter 4.5 mm) were fastened into the femur. The existence of chamfers in the holes of the DCPs, visible in Figure 7.3a, in particular in the inner holes, allows performing the approximation movement of the two fracture lines (Figure 7.3 b). In the final stage of tightening the two inner screws, normal compressive stresses are induced in the interface plane of the two segments (Figure 7.3 c). In effect, the interference of the screw head with the surfaces of the plate chamfer, for a screw placed in the eccentric position (in compression), forces the movement of the bone parts in the convergent direction of the fracture joint. These conditions, which in Orthopaedics correspond to the exercise of a technique known as dynamic compression, correspond to good surgical practice, as they ensure better regeneration of the bone tissue in the fractured region, once the intended reduction

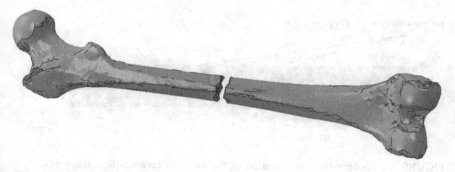

FIGURE 7.1 Transverse fracture.

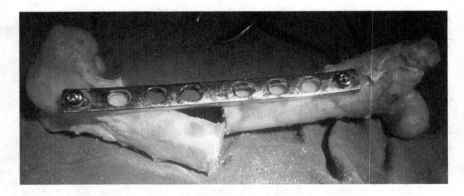

FIGURE 7.2 Transverse fracture of a goat femur and DCP employed for immobilisation.

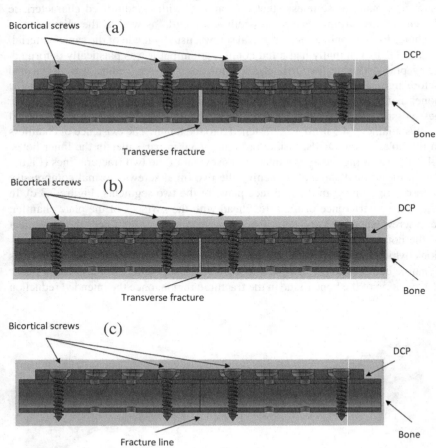

FIGURE 7.3 Schematic representation of the dynamic compression stages aiming to induce compressive stresses in the fracture line.

has been completed. Once the tightening of the two central screws is completed, the remaining ones should be fastened. It should be noted that the screws located in each one of the holes might have different lengths, adjusted to the region of the bone where they are inserted. There is a great diversity of screw lengths, aiming minimising the invasion of the biological tissues surrounding the bone piece since bone does not present a constant section along its length. Figures 7.4a-b show the final assembly of the DCPs performed in the lateral position of the femur, with the corresponding stabilisation of the bone fracture. The overlaps of some screws observed in Figure 7.4b correspond to a measurement less than or equal to 2 mm, which is recommended as the maximum acceptable in this surgical technique.

Subsequently, an experimental setup for four-point bending tests was used (Figure 7.5). A span of 110 mm and a distance of 39 mm between loading cylinders (at the top) were considered. Loading displacement was applied with a rate of

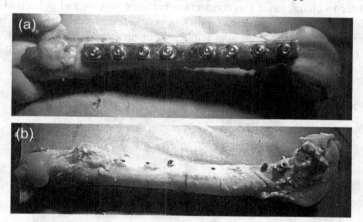

FIGURE 7.4 Fixation of osteosynthesis plate (DCP) by bicortical screws in a transverse fracture; (a) front view and (b) back view.

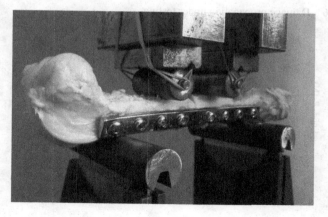

FIGURE 7.5 Experimental setup of the four-point bending test.

0.5 mm/min and the specimen was duly irrigated with physiological saline solution in the course of the test. The test was stopped when the femur fracture was verified, with clear damage propagation (Figure 7.6) reflecting on load decrease (Figure 7.7).

It is observed that generally damage starts in the vicinity of holes as a result of stress concentrations induced by them. The several peaks on the load–displacement curve followed by a decrease of stiffness (Figure 7.7) reflect the successive occurrence of cracks, until the maximum load corresponding to a general failure of the arrangement is attained.

The longitudinal elastic modulus (E_L) of goat cortical bone was obtained from three-point bending tests (Section 2.2) on beam-shaped specimens, taking into account Eq. (2.8) and the following dimensions (in mm): $2L = 55$, $2h = 7.5$, $B = 2$. The overall elastic properties of goat cortical bone tissue are presented in Table 7.1.

In order to characterise the connection between screws and holes and determine the respective cohesive law, pull-out screw tests were performed in four shaft sections harvested from goat femurs. Four identical bone samples (30 mm in length each) were obtained from three osteotomies executed in the diaphysis

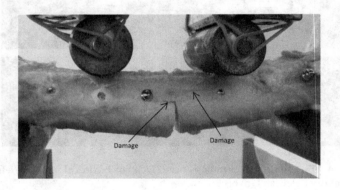

FIGURE 7.6   Damage propagation under testing.

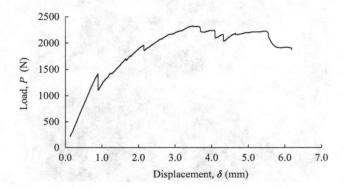

FIGURE 7.7   Load–displacement curve of the four-point bending test.

TABLE 7.1

Elastic Properties of Goat Cortical Bone Tissue

E_L	10,000 MPa
$E_R = E_T$	8,900 MPa[a]
$\upsilon_{LT} = \upsilon_{LR}$	0.17[b]
υ_{RT}	0.18[b]
G_{RT}	3,600 MPa[b]
$G_{RL} = G_{LT}$	3,570 MPa[b]

[a]From B. Pereira et al. (2018); [b]from Patil et al. (2020).

region. Each sample was then radially drilled in the central section and thread-milled. Cortical screws (nominal diameter of 4.5 mm) were subsequently fastened through the cortical wall and bone marrow. During the tests, specimens were fixed to a metal plate fastened to a base (Figure 7.8a). The bicortical screw was pulled out by its head, which was fixed to a steel U-profile and a dowel (Figure 7.8b).

The followed experimental procedure guarantees that the energy is dissipated in the form of damage in the bone-threaded region, thus allowing to characterise the connection at the bone–screw interface. Figure 7.9 presents the load–displacement curves of four pull-out tests. Despite some scatter, typical of natural materials, coherent trends can be found. Specimens harvested from the femoral extremities (1 and 4 in Figure 7.9) reveal higher values of initial stiffness and pull-out strength, which is explained by the circumstance that bone thickness in those regions tends to increase, which is also followed by the rise of trabecular bone.

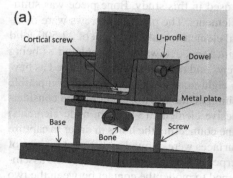
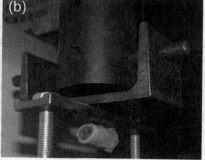

FIGURE 7.8   Schematic representation (a) and pull-out test (b) in goat cortical bone.

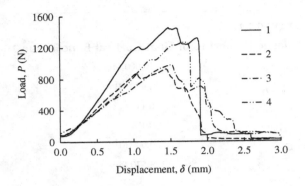

FIGURE 7.9   Load–displacement curves obtained in pull-out tests.

7.1.2   NUMERICAL ANALYSIS

A finite element analysis including cohesive zone modelling of the experimental setup was performed. The main goal was to evaluate the stress field and identify the critical regions prone to damage development.

The numerical model was constructed following several steps. Initially, the tested specimen was cross-sectioned in several planes aiming to identify the geometry of the irregularly shaped bone piece with great accuracy, but also the position of the screws placed along the femur. The three-dimensional mesh was based on the successive arrangement (in space) of all the two-dimensional contours previously collected by photographic registration, from the series of cross-sections, with the same distance at which they were collected. The images were subsequently exported to solid modelling software, which allowed modelling of the bone piece (Figure 7.10).

During the assembly, the osteosynthesis plate was plastically deformed to adjust to the geometric configuration of the bone. Consequently, in the solid modelling phase, it was decided to design/build the plate above the surface of the bone model. This ensured that the osteosynthesis plate could be compatible with the morphology of the bone specimen used in this study. Bone piece was simulated by 11,788 eight-node brick solid elements. The plate and screws were modelled by eight-node brick and tetrahedral elements, making a total of 22,500 solid elements. For the sake of model simplification, screws were simulated as being smooth without fillets. Thereby, the screws and the holes were considered as having the same diameter (3 mm) and 256 eight-node cohesive elements compatible with the solid brick ones were used to simulate the tearing phenomenon considering an appropriate softening law. Cohesive elements (348 eight-node elements) were also inserted in the meridional plane connecting the holes in order to capture the observed fracture profile. Contact surfaces were defined in different regions of the finite element mesh to avoid the interpenetration of various parts of the assembly. The generation of these surfaces aimed to model the contact between the two bone pieces, the interference between the screw heads and the plate chamfers and

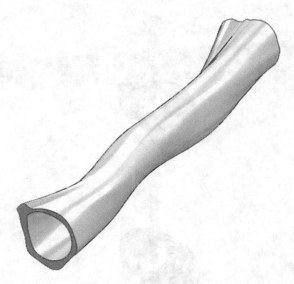

FIGURE 7.10 Final configuration of the bone piece.

the contact between the bone surface and the DCPs. Figure 7.11 presents a global view of the finite element mesh used for the simulations.

In order to determine the cohesive parameters of the screw–bone interaction, an inverse procedure involving the finite element method with cohesive zone analysis was applied in the context of pull-out tests (Figure 7.12).

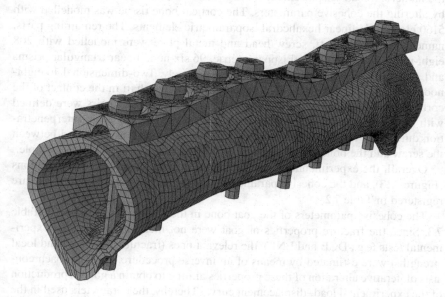

FIGURE 7.11 Global view of the used finite element mesh.

(a)

(b)

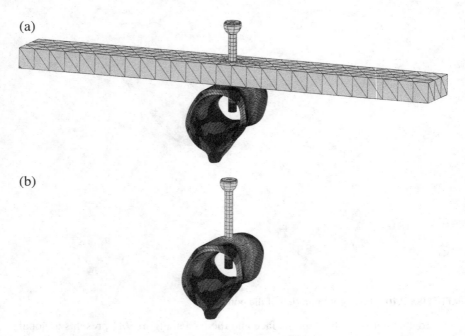

FIGURE 7.12 Numerical simulation of pull-out tests: (a) global setup and (b) detail of deformation in the vicinity of the hole.

The methodology consists of an iterative inverse approach based on fitting the numerical load–displacement curve with the experimental one for each case, by altering the cohesive parameters. The cortical bone tissue was modelled with 5160 eight-node linear hexahedral isoparametric elements. The remaining parts, namely the screw shaft, screw head and metal plate were modelled with 208 eight-node linear hexahedral isoparametric, 96 six-node linear triangular prisms and 1320 four-node tetrahedral element, respectively. Two-dimensional 16 eight-node cohesive elements were disposed along the screw shaft in the contact of the cortical bone to simulate the screw–bone interface. Contact pairs were defined with rigid interaction between the screw and metal plate to avoid interpenetration during the loading process, while softening contact was modelled between the screw and the bone sample, as well as with the metal plate and bone sample.

Overall, the experimental curves were well reproduced after some iterations (Figure 7.13), and the cohesive parameters leading to the observed agreement are registered in Table 7.2.

The cohesive parameters of the goat bone in the TL system are listed in Table 7.3. Since the fracture properties of goat were not measured in specific experimental tests (e.g., DCB and ENF), the relevant ones (fracture toughness and local strengths) were estimated by means of an inverse procedure. This approach consists of iterative alteration of these properties aiming to obtain a good reproduction of the experimental load–displacement curve. Thereby, the parameters used in the

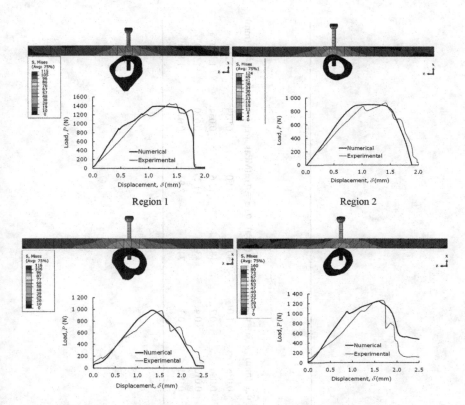

FIGURE 7.13 Experimental and numerical curves of pull-out tests.

cohesive elements located in the bone piece to simulate the longitudinal cracks developing under the four-point bending tests are the ones listed in Table 7.3.

The profile of longitudinal normal stresses induced by loading bending is shown in Figure 7.14a for the entire specimen and, in more detail, for the fractured region in Figure 7.14b. A special remark for the stress concentration effects close to the holes, which explain the origin of the cracks in these regions. Figure 7.15 plots the shear stress distributions, where it is also visible that regions around the screws are the most critical ones. These aspects led to the conclusion that choosing an osteosynthesis plate with the positions of the screw axes arranged along a line tends to reduce significantly the mechanical strength of the connection, as they potentiate the installation of high-tension gradients along the same plane.

Figure 7.16 shows the damage propagation obtained numerically that compares well with the experimental one (Figure 7.6). As discussed above, fracture tends to follow the line of the holes connecting the several stress concentration points.

Figure 7.17 shows a comparison of the numerical load–displacement curve with the experimental one. It can be seen that the numerical model reproduces well the initial stiffness of the assembly and the first peak of load corresponding to an imposed displacement approximately equal to 1 mm. This point corresponds

TABLE 7.2
Cohesive Parameters Obtained in Pull-out Tests

Sec.	G_{Ic} (N/mm)	$G_{IIIc} = G_{IIc}$ (N/mm)	$\sigma_{1,I}$ (MPa)	$\sigma_{1,III} = \sigma_{1,II}$(MPa)	$\delta_{2,I}$ (mm)	$\delta_{2,III} = \delta_{2,II}$ (mm)	$\sigma_{3,I}$ (MPa)	$\sigma_{3,III} = \sigma_{3,II}$(MPa)	$\delta_{3,I}$ (mm)	$\delta_{3,III} = \delta_{3,II}$ (mm)
1	2.00	70.0	50.0	60	0.035	1.0	30.10	24.0	0.039	1.200
2	1.63	45.0	29.3	35	0.050	0.7	18.83	12.6	0.054	1.450
3	1.63	35.0	70.0	33	0.010	0.4	43.73	11.27	0.020	1.270
4	1.63	41.3	110.0	30	0.001	0.1	74.32	8.97	0.010	1.890

TABLE 7.3
Cohesive Parameters for Goat Cortical Bone in the TL System

G_{Ic} (N/mm)	$G_{IIc} = G_{IIIc}$ (N/mm)	$\sigma_{1,I}$ (MPa)	$\sigma_{1,III} = \sigma_{1,II}$ (MPa)	$\delta_{2,I}$ (mm)	$\delta_{2,III} = \delta_{2,II}$ (mm)	$\sigma_{3,I}$ (MPa)	$\sigma_{3,III} = \sigma_{3,II}$ (MPa)	$\delta_{3,I}$ (mm)	$\delta_{3,III} = \delta_{3,II}$ (mm)
1.5	2.0	20.0	20.0	0.01	0.01	10.0	10.0	0.075	0.1

(a)

(b)

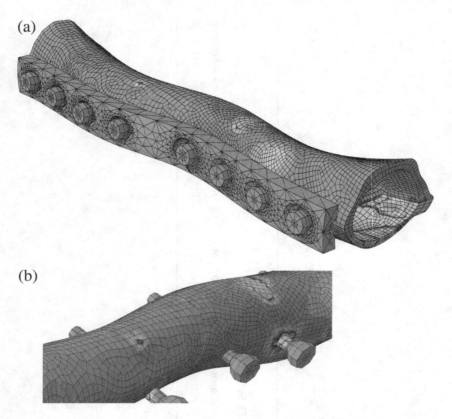

FIGURE 7.14 Longitudinal normal stresses (a) for the entire specimen and (b) detail of the region close to the fracture surface.

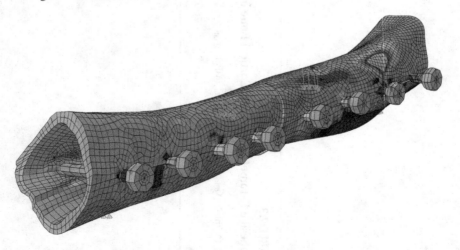

FIGURE 7.15 Shear stresses profile for the entire specimen.

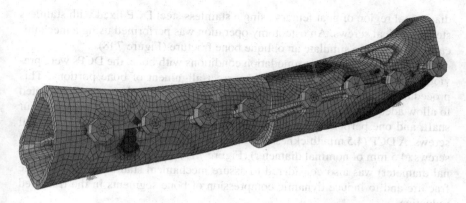

FIGURE 7.16 Damage propagation obtained numerically.

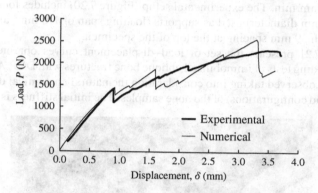

FIGURE 7.17 Numerical and experimental load–displacement curves of the transverse fracture.

to the first damage propagation and can be viewed as the design strength of the assembly. Anyway, beyond this point, it can be stated that the numerical curve overall describes the experimental tendency, which proves that the proposed methodology can be regarded as a valuable tool to predict the mechanical and fracture behaviour of the repair of the bone transverse fracture.

7.2 OBLIQUE FRACTURE

7.2.1 EXPERIMENTAL TESTS

Oblique fracture occurs frequently because of shear and bending loading and is conditioned by the internal microstructural arrangement of bone. It is characterised by a fracture plane oblique to the longitudinal bone axis and it is more complex to immobilise than the transverse one.

This study carried out an experimental characterisation and numerical analysis of an immobilisation system of an oblique fracture, located in the central diaphyseal region of goat femurs using a stainless steel DCP fixed with stainless steel bicortical screws. An osteotomy operation was performed using a mechanical saw in order to simulate an oblique bone fracture (Figure 7.18).

Aiming to increase accommodation conditions with bone, the DCPs were previously deformed thus providing the correct alignment of bone portions. This procedure has been executed following the surgical protocols currently executed to allow adequate bone repair. Six threaded holes were executed along the femur shaft, and one perpendicularly to the central oblique fracture to fasten cortical screws. A DCP (4.5 mm thickness) with staggered holes was fixed using bicortical screws (4.5 mm of nominal diameter) (Figure 7.19). A *Lag* screw (3 mm of nominal diameter) was also considered to assure mechanical stabilisation of oblique fracture and to induce dynamic compression of bone segments in the fractured reduction.

Four 4-point bending tests were performed under displacement control with a rate of 0.5 mm/min. The experimental setup (Figure 7.20) includes four steel cylinders (10 mm diameter) used as supports (loading span of 110 mm) and loading devices with 39 mm spacing at the top of the specimen.

Figure 7.21 presents the set of load–displacement curves obtained in four 4-point bending tests of immobilised oblique bone fractures with DCP. Acceptable scatter was observed taking into consideration the natural anatomical differences (i.e., size and configurations) of the bone samples. The initial stiffness is consistent

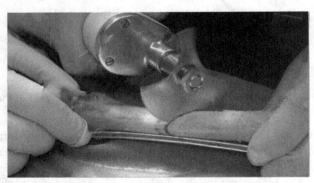

FIGURE 7.18   Cutting operation to simulate an oblique fracture.

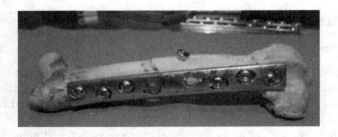

FIGURE 7.19   Fixation of DCP and *Lag* screw to the femur shaft.

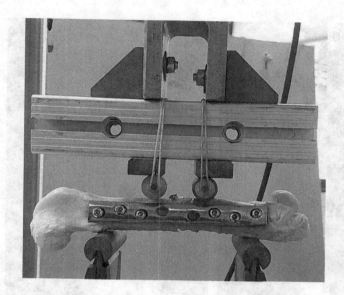

FIGURE 7.20 Experimental setup used for the four-point bending tests.

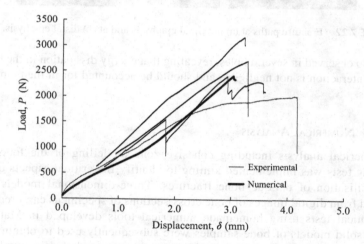

FIGURE 7.21 Load–displacement curves of the four-point bending tests for the oblique fracture.

among the tested specimens. The observed sudden drops in the applied load are explained by crack propagation occurring near the screws used to fasten the metal plate. Examination of bone samples after testing revealed that cracks consistently initiated near the fracture line (central oblique fracture) and propagated in the direction of the first hole (Figure 7.22). This statement is a consequence of stress concentration effects around these regions. The crack paths in bone (Figure 7.22 a, b) were marked with ink, thus providing better visualisation. Screw loosening

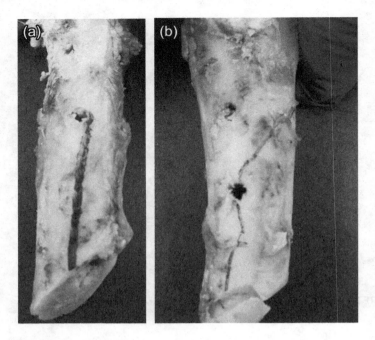

FIGURE 7.22   Fracture paths at (a) proximal epiphysis and at (b) distal epiphysis.

was also observed in several holes, revealing that energy dissipation in the bone–
screw interaction is not negligible and should be accounted for in the numerical
analysis.

7.2.2 Numerical Analysis

A numerical analysis including cohesive zone modelling of the four-point
bending tests was implemented aiming to identify the critical aspects of this
immobilisation of oblique bone fractures. Three-dimensional models were
defined from digital images of bone cross-sections of specimens captured after
mechanical tests using homemade numerical tools developed in MatLab®.
These solid models of bone samples were subsequently used to obtain finite
element meshes (Figure 7.23a). The bone shaft was modelled in two halves
with 133,536 six-node linear triangular prism elements, while the DCP and
the four cylinders were modelled with 77,222 four-node tetrahedral elements
and 576 eight-node brick elements, respectively. The bicortical screws (six to
fasten the plate and one for the *Lag*) were modelled in the same way as for
the pull-out screw tests. Two types of six-node cohesive elements compatible
with the employed solid elements were used in this analysis. For the interfaces
of screw–cortical bone, a total of 765 cohesive elements with null thickness
were disposed along the screw shafts of 7 bicortical screws, while 548 six-
node cohesive elements were included in the bone shaft to simulate damage

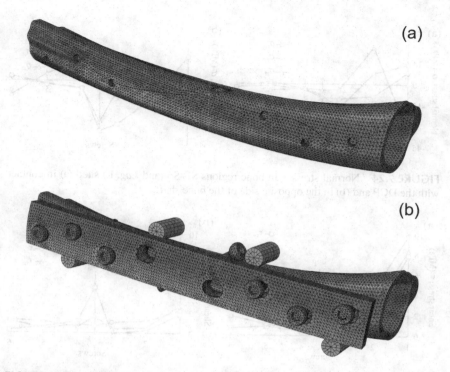

FIGURE 7.23   Finite element mesh (a) of the bone shaft and (b) the four-point bending tests (inscriptions S1-S6 and L refer to the screws).

initiation and propagation in the vicinity of the screw holes. Contact surfaces were also considered in all interactions (i.e., plate–bone shaft, screws–plate, cylinders–bone shaft) to prevent unwanted interpenetration in the course of the loading process. The numerical model of the four-point bending testing setup is shown in Figure 7.23b.

The load was applied under displacement control considering small increments (0.5% of the applied displacement) to induce stable damage propagation. Boundary conditions were applied in agreement with the experiments and a non-linear geometrical analysis was considered.

A preliminary stress analysis was performed aiming to identify the critical points of the assembly. The normal and shear stress profiles in the regions close to screws (S1 to S6 and *Lag*, L) at each side of the bone shaft (i.e., in contact with the DCP and on the opposite side) are presented in Figures 7.24 and 7.25. Peak values of normal (Figure. 7.24a, b) and shear stresses (Figure 7.25a, b) have been registered for screw S1. The region affected by the *Lag* screw (L) can also be regarded as a critical point of this reinforcement system. Overall, Figures 7.25 and 7.26 prove that relevant stress concentration effects take place close to the bolted joints of cortical bone revealing important variation along the bone shaft when submitted to bending.

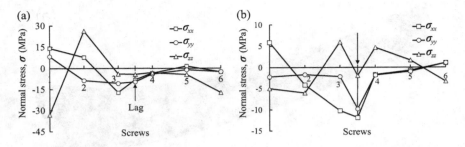

FIGURE 7.24 Normal stresses in bone regions S1–S6 (and *Lag*, L) sited (a) in contact with the DCP and (b) in the opposite side of the bone shaft.

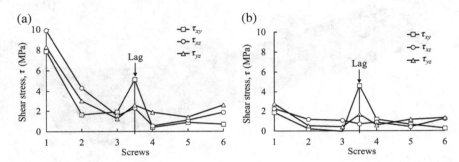

FIGURE 7.25 Shear stress in bone regions S1–S6 (and Lag, L) sited (a) in contact with the DCP and (b) in the opposite side of the bone shaft.

A stress analysis of the oblique fracture section and the *Lag* screw was also performed considering the von Mises stresses (Figure 7.26). Although the *Lag* screw reveals the maximum stress values in the vicinity of the fracture section, it can be observed that for the induced bending loading the lower part of the oblique fracture section is almost under quite small or even null stresses. Since bone healing requires the existence of compressive stresses at the fracture section, it can be settled that this is a critical region regarding the bone healing process.

The progressive damage analysis of the bone repair under four-point bending was performed considering the cohesive and elastic properties used in Section 7.1. In Figure 7.27, the DCP was removed in order to show the crack path propagation obtained numerically. As observed experimentally, cracks have propagated due to stress concentration effects occurring in regions near the drill holes (Figure 7.27). The developed model was able to mimic both the screw loosening phenomenon and crack development in the vicinity of screws.

The numerical load–displacement curve of the four-point bending test was also included in Figure 7.21 for the sake of comparison with the experimental ones. Overall, it can be settled that global experimental trends are well captured. In fact, the initial stiffness and the loading peak are adequately reproduced. It can be concluded that the numerical model including cohesive zone analysis is a

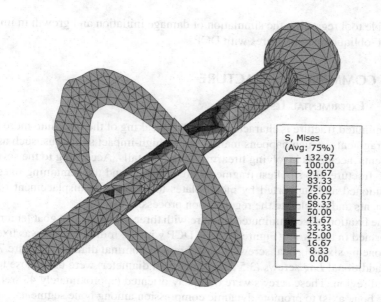

FIGURE 7.26 von Mises stress distribution (MPa) at the *Lag* (L) screw and at the oblique fracture surface.

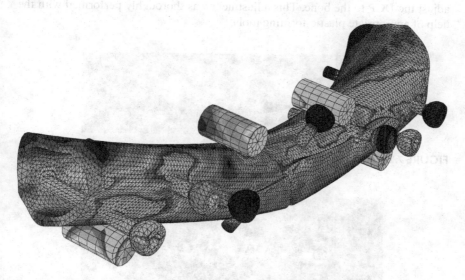

FIGURE 7.27 Crack path obtained numerically for the four-point bending test.

valuable tool regarding the simulation of damage initiation and growth in immobilised oblique bone fractures with DCP.

7.3 COMMINUTED FRACTURE

7.3.1 EXPERIMENTAL TESTS

Comminuted fracture is characterised by the breaking of the bone into more than two fragments, which happens mainly due to high-impact situations, such as car accidents, accidents involving firearms or serious falls. According to the severity of the fracture, the smallest fragments are removed and the remaining ones are repositioned and supported by metal plates to prevent the displacement of the fragments and accelerate the regeneration process.

The fixation of a comminuted fracture with three segments in a goat femur was performed in this work (Figure 7.28). A DCP with 4.5 mm thickness was fixed to the bone by six bicortical screws with 4.5 mm of nominal diameter (Figure 7.29). Two additional *Lag* screws (3.5 mm of nominal diameter) were used close to the central region. These screws were obliquely oriented (approximately 45° relative to the bone axis) to promote dynamic compression among bone segments.

Figure 7.30 reveals the final assembly showing the proximity of the heads of the two *Lag* screws differently oriented (approximately 90° between them), as well as the end of the plate fixation screws (about 2 mm), following Orthopaedics recommendations. Before performing the mechanical test, it was necessary to adjust the DCP to the bone. This adjustment was thoroughly performed with the help of appropriate plastic-forming tools.

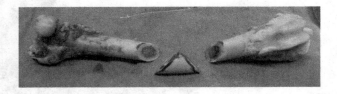

FIGURE 7.28 Comminuted fracture with three segments.

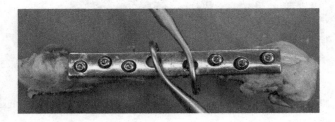

FIGURE 7.29 Assembly illustrating the six bicortical screws used to fix the DCP to bone.

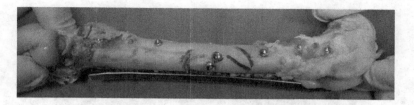

FIGURE 7.30 Final assembly bone/DCP for a comminuted fracture.

As in previous cases, the four-point bending test was used to assess the mechanical and fracture behaviour of the employed assembly. The distance between support cylinders (10 mm diameter) was set to 110 mm, while the distance between the load application cylinders (10 mm diameter) was set to 39 mm. These dimensions were revealed to comply with a strategy to make maximum use of the femoral diaphysis length, and of the central region surface that would prevent interference with the *Lag* screws. The test (Figure 7.31, b) was performed with a displacement rate of 0.5 mm/min with a maximum prescribed displacement of 15 mm.

The experimental test was stopped when visible fractures occurred in the bone (Figure 7.32). These fractures are located in the centre of one of the holes with extension/projection towards the extremity that is in contact with the fracture line that was produced with the mechanical saw. In the four-point bending configuration, shear stresses develop in the regions between the supports and the load application points. Thus, it can be stated that the location of this damage in the region between the supports and the load application points is coherent, as it occurs in

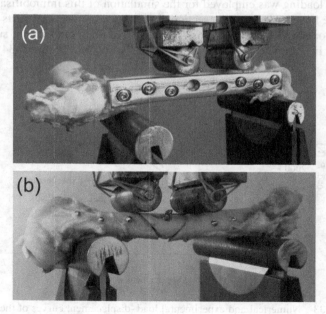

FIGURE 7.31 Experimental test setup; a) front view; b) back view.

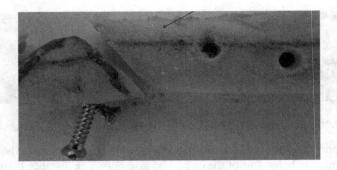

FIGURE 7.32 Occurrence of fractures (identified by an arrow) in bone.

a region with high concentration of stresses (due to bolts) and shear stresses due to bending.

The ensuing experimental load–displacement curve (Figure 7.33) reveals two different regions. An initial almost linear branch up to 3000 N, approximately, followed by a clear stiffness reduction in the range of 5–6 mm of applied displacement. The first part reflects the initial stiffness of the assembly and the second one is a consequence of the damage development identified in Figure 7.32.

7.3.2 NUMERICAL ANALYSIS

The developed numerical model including cohesive zone analysis with mixed-mode I+II loading was employed for the simulation of this immobilisation technique. The bone specimen was sectioned transversely in several parts to enable rigorous bone modelling. The cross-sections were photographed for subsequent treatment in computed-aided design (CAD) software (Figure 7.34). In this

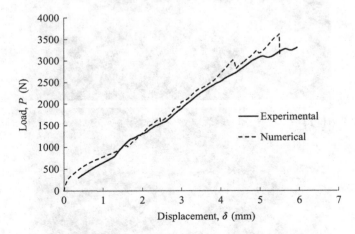

FIGURE 7.33 Numerical and experimental load–displacement curves of the four-point bending test.

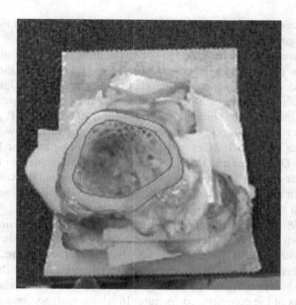

FIGURE 7.34 Outer and inner contours of the cortical bone in one part of the bone piece.

software, the exterior and interior contours of each cut were defined aiming to generate the three-dimensional model of the bone pieces.

Once this task was completed, the bone piece was reassembled in order to take photographs for subsequent treatment in the CAD software. As a result of these operations, the solid model of the entire (Figure 7.35a) and fractured femur (Figure 7.35b) was built. Similar procedures were followed to obtain the solid

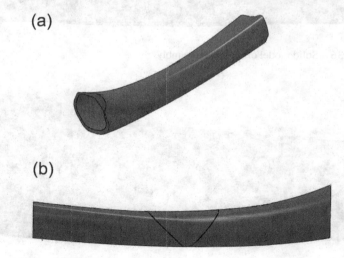

FIGURE 7.35 Solid model of the entire (a) and fractured femur (b).

models for the screws and for the DCP, thus allowing getting the final assembly modelled (Figure 7.36).

The solid models were then used to obtain the finite element mesh employed in the simulation of the mechanical test. Owing to its geometry, the inner bone part was modelled with four-node solid tetrahedral elements while eight-node solid hexahedral elements were considered in the outer ones. These types of elements were also employed in the simulation of the screws and of the DCP, giving rise to a total number of 19,414 solid elements. Several contact surfaces were defined to avoid spurious interpenetrations between the three bone parts, the DCP and the bone and the DCP holes and the screw heads. Cohesive elements of eight nodes were considered in the region prone to crack propagation and between the screws and bone for a total of 396 elements. The goal was to simulate damage initiation and growth at these critical regions (Figure 7.37).

Figure 7.38 illustrates the normal stress field installed in the direction of the bone piece axis for 50% of the total applied displacement. This stress state results from the transmission of the efforts applied directly on the bone piece, which are transferred through the screws, to the plate. The discontinuity of the stress field observed in the upper region of the femur model is due to the existence of two fracture joints of the comminuted fracture. In addition, stress concentrations can also be observed in the vicinity of screws. The cracks developed in the model are illustrated in Figure 7.39, as well as the detachment of the screws near the holes, which proves the robustness of the numerical model.

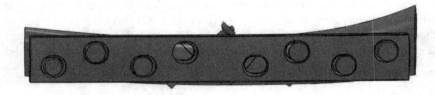

FIGURE 7.36　Solid model of the final assembly.

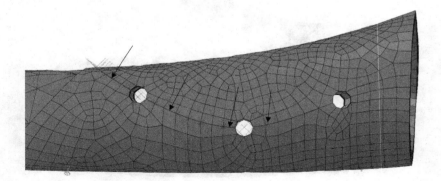

FIGURE 7.37　Location of the cohesive elements (identified by the arrows).

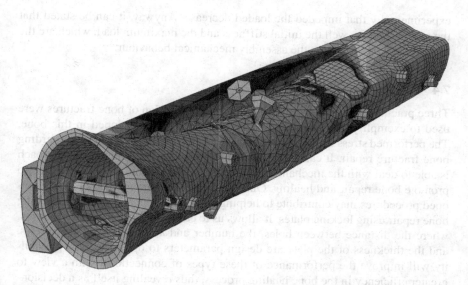

FIGURE 7.38   Normal stress field along the longitudinal bone axis.

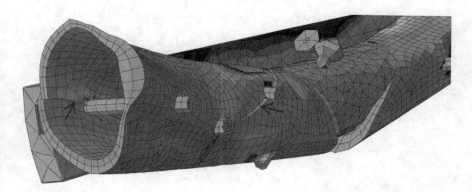

FIGURE 7.39   Detail illustrating the cracks developed in the model (identified by the arrows).

The numerical load–displacement curve is compared with the experimental one in Figure 7.33. Overall, it can be stated that the numerical curve follows the experimental one. The initial stiffness of the assembly is well captured. The small peaks reflect damage development at the several sites identified in Figure 7.39. By the end, the numerical curve exhibits a peak load close to the maximum experimental value followed by an abrupt decrease not observed experimentally. The reason behind such difference relies on the contact occurring between the loading cylinders with the DCP after pronounced damage development observed experimentally that impeded the loaded decrease. Anyway, it can be stated that the model captures well the initial stiffness and the maximum load, which are the main parameters to assess the assembly mechanical behaviour.

7.4   CLOSING REMARKS

Three practical applications involving the immobilisation of bone fractures were used to exemplify the usefulness of the methodologies developed in this bone. The performed stress and progressive damage analyses are crucial tools regarding bone fracture repair. It can be concluded that the proposed numerical approach is able to deal with the mechanical behaviour of the assemblies typically used to promote bone repair and healing. Once applied to human bone tissue, the developed procedures may contribute to helping surgeons support decisions regarding bone repair using locking plates. It allows us to easily study alternative scenarios, where the distance between holes, the number and arrangement of the screws, and the thickness of the plate are design parameters to optimise. This possibility will improve the performance of these types of connections, with a view to greater efficiency in the bone healing process, thus revealing itself as a decision-supporting tool for orthopaedic teams in the surgical context.

References

Acevedo C, Stadelmann VA, Pioletti DP, 2018. Fatigue as the missing link between bone fragility and fracture. *Nat Biomed Eng* 2:62–71.

Adachi E, Hopkinson I, Hayashi T, 1997. Basement–membrane stromal relationships: Interactions between collagen fibrils and the lamina densa. *Int Rev Cytol* 173:73–156.

Akhter MP, Wells DJ, Short SJ, Cullen DM, Johnson ML, Haynatzki GR, Babij P, Allen KM, Yaworsky PJ, Bex F, Recker R, 2004. Bone biomechanical properties in LRP5 mutant mice. *Bone* 35:162–169.

Akkus O, Jepsen KJ, Rimnac CM, 2000. Microstructural aspects of the fracture process in human cortical bone. *J Mater Sc* 35:6065–6074.

Aliha MRM, Mousavi SS, 2020. Sub-sized short bend beam configuration for the study of mixed-mode fracture. *Eng Fract Mech* 225:106830.

Anderson C, 1995. Molecular biology of matrix vesicles. *Clin Orthop Relat Res* 314:266–280.

Ashman RB, Cowin SC, Van Buskirk WC, Rice JC, 1984. Continuous wave technique for the measurement of the elastic properties of cortical bone. *J Biomechanics* 17:349–361.

ASTM standard D5379/D5379M – 12. 2012. *Standard test method for shear properties of composite materials by the V-notched beam method.* ASTM International, West Conshohocken, PA, www.astm.org.

ASTM standard D7078/D7078M – 12. 2012. *Standard test method for shear properties of composite materials by v-notched rail shear method.* ASTM International, West Conshohocken, PA, www.astm.org.

Banerjee J, Azevedo HS, 2017. Crafting of functional biomaterials by directed molecular self-assembly of triple helical peptide building blocks. *Interface Focus* 7:20160138.

Behiri JC, Bonfield W, 1989. Orientation dependence of the fracture mechanics of cortical bone. *J Biomech* 22:863–872.

Boivin G, 2007. The hydroxyapatite crystal: A closer look. *Medicographia* 29:126–132.

Bonewald LF, Johnson ML, 2008. Osteocytes, mechanosensing and Wnt signaling. *Bone* 42:606–615.

Bonnet N, Bernard P, Beaupied H, Bizot JC, Trovero F, Courteix D, Benhamou CL, 2007. Various effects of antidepressant drugs on bone microarchitecture, mechanical properties and bone remodeling. *Toxicol Appl Pharmacol* 221:111–118.

Boskey AL, Robey PG, 2013. The regulatory role of matrix proteins in mineralization of bone in osteoporosis. In: Marcus R, Feldman D, Dempster DW, Luckey M, Cauley JA (Eds.), *Osteoporosis.* Academic Press, Cambridge, 235–255.

Bowman SM, Gibson LJ, Hayes WC, McMahon TA, 1999. Results from demineralized bone creep tests suggest that collagen is responsible for the creep behaviour of bone. *J Biomech Eng* 121:253–258.

Bozec L, van der Heijden G, Horton M, 2007. Collagen fibrils: Nanoscale ropes. *Biophys J* 92:70–75.

Brown CU, Yeni YN, Norman TL, 2000. Fracture toughness is dependent on bone location - A study of the femoral neck, femoral shaft, and the tibial shaft. *J Biomedical Mater Res* 49:380–389.

Brown JL, Laurencin CT, 2020. Bone tissue engineering. In: Wagner WR, Sakiyama-Elbert SE, Zhang G, Yaszemski MJ (Eds.), *Biomaterials science* (4th Edition). Academic Press, Cambridge, MA, 1373–1388.

Buehler MJ, Wong SY, 2007. Entropic elasticity controls nanomechanics of single tropocollagen molecules. *Biophys J* 93:37–43.

Burger C, Zhou HW, Wang H, Sics I, Hsiao BS, Chu B, Graham L, Glimcher MJ, 2008. Lateral packing of mineral crystals in bone collagen fibrils. *Biophys J* 95:1985–1992.

Burr DB, Forwood MR, Fyhrie DP, Martin RB, Schaffler MB, Turner CH, 1997. Bone microdamage and skeletal fragility in osteoporotic and stress fractures. *J Bone Miner Res* 12:6–15.

Burr DB, Schaffler MB, Frederickson RG, 1988. Composition of the cement line and its possible mechanical role as a local interface in human compact bone. *J Biomech* 21:939–945.

Campo RD, Romano JE, 1986. Changes in cartilage proteoglycans associated with calcification. *Calcif Tissue Int* 39:175–184.

Carter DR, Caler WE, 1983. Cycle-dependent and time-dependent bone fracture with repeated loading. *J Biomech Eng* 105:166–170.

Carter DR, Hayes WC, 1977. Compact bone fatigue damage: A microscopic examination. *CORR* 127:265–274.

Cezayirlioglu H, Bahniuk E, Davy DT, Heiple KG, 1985. Anisotropic yield behavior of bone under combined axial force and torque. *J Biomech* 18:61–69.

Clarke B, 2008. Normal bone anatomy and physiology. *Clin J Am Soc Nephrol* 3 Suppl 3:131–139.

Cowin SC, 1986. Fabric dependence of an anisotropic strength criterion. *Mech Mater* 5:251–260.

Cowin SC, 2001. *Bone mechanics handbook* (2nd edition). CRC Press, New York.

Currey JD, 1988a. The effect of porosity and mineral content on the Young's modulus of elasticity of compact bone. *J Biomech* 21:131–139.

Currey JD, 1988b. The effects of drying and re-wetting on some mechanical properties of cortical bone. *J Biomech* 5:439–441.

Currey JD, 2002. *Bones: Structure and Mechanics*. Princeton University Press, Princeton, NJ.

de Moura MFSF, Cavaleiro PMLC, Silva FGA, Dourado N, 2017. Mixed-mode I+II fracture characterization of a hybrid carbon-epoxy/cork laminate using the single-leg bending test. *Compos Sci Technol* 141:24–31.

de Moura MFSF, Dourado N, Morais JJL, Pereira FAM, 2010. Numerical analysis of the ENF and ELS tests applied to mode II fracture characterization of cortical bone tissue. *Fat Fract Eng Mater Struct* 34:149–158.

de Moura MFSF, Gonçalves JPM, 2014. Cohesive zone model for high-cycle fatigue of adhesively bonded joints under mode I loading. *Int J Solids Struct* 51:1123–1131.

de Moura MFSF, Gonçalves JPM, 2015. Cohesive zone model for high-cycle fatigue of composite bonded joints under mixed-mode I+II loading. *Eng Fract Mech* 140:31–42.

de Moura MFSF, Gonçalves JPM, Silva FGA, 2016. A new energy based mixed-mode cohesive zone model. *Int J Solids Struct* 102–103:112–119.

Doerner MF, Nix WD, 1986. A method for interpreting the data from depth-sensing indentation instruments. *J Mater Res* 1:601–609.

Dong XN, Guo XE, 2000. Is the cement line a weak interface? Paper 0036 of the 46th Annual Meeting, Orthopaedic Research Society, March 12–15, 2000, Orlando, Florida.

Donough MJ, Gunnion AJ, Orifici AC, Wang CH, 2015. Plasticity induced crack closure in adhesively bonded joints under fatigue loading. *Int J Fatigue* 70:440–450.

Dourado N, Pereira FAM, de Moura MFSF, Morais JJL, Dias MIR, 2013. Bone fracture characterization using the end notched flexure test. *Mater Sc Eng C* 33:405–410.

Dziewaitkowski DD, Majznerski LL, 1985. Role of proteoglycans in endochondral ossification: Inhibition of calcification. *Calcif Tissue Int* 37:560–564.

Farokhi M et al., 2018. Silk fibroin/hydroxyapatite composites for bone tissue engineering. *Biotechnol Adv* 36:68–91.

Feng Z, Rho J, Han S, Ziv I, 2000. Orientation and loading condition dependence of fracture toughness in cortical bone. *Mater Sci Eng C* 11:41–46.

Fratzl P, Gupta HS, Paschalis EP, Roschger P, 2004. Structure and mechanical quality of the collagen-mineral nano-composite in bone. *J Mater Chem* 14:2115–2123.

Gautieri A, Buehler MJ, Redaelli A, 2009. Deformation rate controls elasticity and unfolding pathway of single tropocollagen molecules. *J Mech Behav Biomed* 2:130–137.

Gelse K, Poschl E, Aigner T, 2003. *Adv Drug Deliv Rev* 55:1531–1546.

George WT, Vashishth T, 2006. Susceptibility of aging human bone to mixed-mode fracture increases bone fragility. *Bone* 38:105–111.

Glimcher MJ, 1998. The nature of the mineral phase in bone: Biological and clinical implications. In: Avioli LV, SM Krane (Eds.), *Metabolic bone disease and clinically related disorders*. Academic Press, San Diego, CA, 23–50.

Gonçalves JPM, de Moura MFSF, de Castro PMST, Marques AT, 2000. Interface element including point-to-surface constraints for three-dimensional problems with damage propagation. *Eng Computation* 17:28–47.

Gottesman T, Hashin Z, 1980. Analysis of viscoelastic behaviour of bones on the basis of microstructure. *J Biomech* 13:89–96.

Granke M, Makowski AJ, Uppuganti S, Nyman JS, 2016. Prevalent role of porosity and osteonal area over mineralization heterogeneity in the fracture toughness of human cortical bone. *J Biomech* 49:2748–2755.

Guo XE, 2001. Mechanical properties of cortical bone and cancellous bone tissue. In: Cowin SC (Ed.), *Bone mechanics handbook* (2nd Edition). CRC Press, Boca Raton, FL. Pages 10-1–10-23.

Hankinson RL, 1921. Investigation of crushing strength of spruce at varying angles of grain, air force information circular No. 259, U. S. Air Service.

Hayes WC, Wright TM, 1977. An empirical strength theory for compact bone. *Fracture* 3:1173–1179.

He G, Dahl T, Veis A, George A, 2003. Nucleation of apatite crystals in vitro by self-assembled dentin matrix protein 1. *Nat Mater* 2:552–558.

He MY, Turner MR, Evans AG, 1995. Analysis of the double cleavage drilled compression specimen for interface fracture energy measurements over a range of mode mixities. *Acta Metall Mater* 43:3453–3458.

Henriksen K, Neutzsky-Wulff AV, Bonewald LF, Karsdal MA, 2009. Local communication on and within bone controls bone remodelling. *Bone* 44:1026–1033.

Hernandez CJ, Beaupré GS, Keller TS, Carter DR, 2001. The influence of bone volume fraction and ash fraction on bone strength and modulus. *Bone* 29:74–78.

Hillgärtner M, Linka K, Itskov M, 2018. Worm-like chain model extensions for highly stretched tropocollagen molecules. *J Biomech* 80:129–135.

Hunt KD, Dean O'Loughlin V, Fitting W, Adler L, 1998. Ultrasonic determination of the elastic modulus of human cortical bone. *Med Biol Eng Comput* 36:51–56.

Irwin GR, 1957. Analysis of stress and strains near the end of a crack traversing a plate, ASME. *J Appl Mech* 24:361–364.

Irwin GR, Kies JA, 1954. Critical energy rate analysis of fracture strength. *Weld J Res Suppl* 33:193s.

ISO. 2001. 15024: Fibre-reinforced plastic composites – Determination of mode I interlaminar fracture toughness, gic, for unidirectionally reinforced materials.

Jepsen KJ, Davy DT, Krzypow DJ, 1999. The role of the lamellar interface during torsional yielding of human cortical bone. *J Biomech* 32:303–310.

Jonsson U, Ranta H, Stromberg L, 1985. Growth changes of collagen cross-linking, calcium, and water content in bone. *Arch Orthop Traum Su* 104:89–93.

Kameo Y, Masahiro O, Taiji A, 2022. Computational framework for analyzing flow-induced strain on osteocyte as modulated by microenvironment. *JMBBM* 126:105027.

Kaplan FS, Lee WC, Keaveny TM, Boskey A, Einhorn TA, Iannotti JP, 1994. Form and function of bone. In: Simon SP (Ed.), *Orthopedic basic science*. American Academy of Orthopedic Surgeons, Columbus, OH, USA, 127–185.

Kinloch AJ, Wang Y, Williams JG, Yayla P, 1993. The mixed-mode delamination of fibre composite materials. *Comp Sci Techol* 47:225–237.

Koester KJ, Barth HD, Ritchie RO, 2011. Effect of aging on the transverse toughness of human cortical bone: Evaluation by *R*-curves. *J Mech Behavior Biomed Mater* 4:1504–1513.

Kohli N, Ho S, Brown SJ, Sawadkar P, Sharma V, Snow M, García-Gareta E, 2018. Bone remodelling in vitro: Where are we headed? – A review on the current understanding of physiological bone remodelling and inflammation and the strategies for testing biomaterials in vitro. *Bone* 110:38–46.

Kolmann FPF, Côté WA, 1984. *Principles of wood science and technology: Solid wood*. Springer-Verlag, Berlin.

Kopp J, Bonnet M, Renou JP, 1989. Effect of collagen cross-linking on collagen-water interactions (a DSC investigation). *Matrix* 9:443–450.

Krueger R, 2002. The virtual crack closure technique: History, approach and applications, NASA/CR-2002-211628, Icase Report No. 2002-10.

Kruger TE, Miller AH, Godwin AK, Wang J, 2014. Bone sialoprotein and osteopontin in bone metastasis of osteotropic cancers. *Crit Rev Oncol Hematol* 89:330–341.

Kruzic JJ, Kim DK, Koester KJ, Ritchie RO, 2009. Indentation techniques for evaluating the fracture toughness of biomaterials and hard tissues. *J Mech Behav Biomed Mater* 2:384–395.

Kumari S, Panda TK, Pradhan T, 2017. Lysyl oxidase: Its diversity in health and diseases. *Indian J Clin Biochem* 32:134–141.

Lacroix D, 2019. Biomechanical aspects of bone repair. In: Pawelec K, Planell J A (Eds.), Whoodhead publishing series in Biomaterials, *Bone repair biomaterials* (2nd Edition). Elsevier, Duxford, United Kingdom, 53–64.

Landis WJ, 1996. Mineral characterization in calcifying tissues: Atomic, molecular and macromolecular perspectives. *Connect Tissue Res* 34:239–246.

Landis WJ, Hodgens KJ, Arena J, Song MJ, McEwen BF, 1996. Structural relations between collagen and mineral in bone as determined by high voltage electron microscopic tomography. *Microsc Res Tech* 33:192–202.

Lardner TJ, Chakravarthy S, Quinn JD, Ritter JE, 2001. Further analysis of the DCDC specimen with an offset hole. *Int J Fract* 109:227–237.

Lecompte D, Smits A, Bossuyt S, Sol H, Vantomme J, Van Hemelrijck D, Habraken AM, 2006. Quality assessment of speckle patterns for digital image correlation. *Opt Lasers Eng* 44:1132–1145.

LeGeros RZ, 1991. *Calcium phosphate in oral biology and medicine*. Meyers, San Francisco, 98.

Lenthe GH, Voide R, Boyd SK, Müller R, 2008. Tissue modulus calculated from beam theory is biased by bone size and geometry: Implications for the use of three-point bending tests to determine bone tissue modulus. *Bone* 43:717–723.

Levenston ME, Beaupré GS, van der Meulen MCH, 1994. Improved method for analysis of whole bone torsion tests. *J Bone Mineral Res* 9:1459–1465.

Lin J-P, Shi Z-J, Shen N-J, Wang J, Li Z-M, Xiao J, 2016. N-terminal telopeptides of type I collagen and bone mineral density for early diagnosis of nonunion: An experimental study in rabbits. *Indian J Orthop* 50:421–426.

Liu JY, 1984. Evaluation of the tensor polynomial strength theory of wood. *J Comp Mat* 18:216–226.

Liu X, Zheng C, Luo X, Wang X, Jiang H, 2019. Recent advances of collagen-based biomaterials: Multi-hierarchical structure, modification and biomedical applications. *Mat Sci Eng C-Mater* 99:1509–1522.

Liu Y, Luo D, Wang T, 2016. Hierarchical structures of bone and bioinspired bone tissue engineering. *Small* 12:4611–4632.

Lowenstam, HA, Weiner S, 1989. *On biomineralization*. Oxford University Press, UK. ISBN 0-19-504977-2.

MacLeod AR, Pankaj P, Simpson AHRW 2012. Does screw–bone interface modelling matter in finite element analyses? *J Biomech* 45:1712–1716.

Mak AFT, Zhang JD, 2001. Numerical simulation of streaming potentials due to deformation-induced hierarchical flows in cortical bone. *J Biomech Eng* 123:66–70.

Martin RB, 2003. Fatigue damage, remodelling and the minimization of skeletal weight. *J Theoret Biology* 220:271–276.

Mecholsky JrJJ, Clifton KB, 2007. How tough is bone? Application of elastic–plastic fracture mechanics to bone. *Bone* 40:479–484.

Morais JJL, de Moura MFSF, Pereira FAM, Xavier JMC, Dourado N, Dias MIR, Azevedo JMT, 2010. The double cantilever beam test applied to mode I fracture characterization of cortical bone tissue. *J Mech Behavior of Biomedical Mater* 3:446–453.

Moreira RDF, de Moura MFSF, Figueiredo MAV, Fernandes RL, 2015. Characterisation of composite bonded single-strap repairs under fatigue loading. *Int J Mech Sci* 103:22–29.

Moreira RDF, de Moura MFSF, Silva FGA, 2020. A novel strategy to obtain the fracture envelope under mixed-mode I+II loading of composite bonded joints. *Eng Fract Mech* 232:107032.

Morgan EF, Barnes GF, Einhorn TA, 2013. The bone organ system: Form and function. In: Marcus R, Feldman D, Dempster DW, Luckey M, Cauley JA (Eds.), *Osteoporosis* vol 1 (4th Edition). Elsevier, London, UK, 3–20.

Nalla RK, Kinney JH, Ritchie RO, 2003. Mechanistic fracture criteria for the failure of human cortical bone. *Nature Mater* 2:164–168.

Nalla RK, Kruzic JJ, Ritchie RO, 2004. On the origin of the toughness of mineralized tissue: Microcracking or crack bridging? *Bone* 34:790–798.

Norman TL, Nivargikar SV, Burr DB, 1996. Resistance to crack growth in human cortical bone is greater in shear than in tension. *J Biomech* 29:1023–1031.

Norman TL, Vashishth D, Burr DB, 1995. Fracture toughness of human bone under tension. *J Biomech* 28:309–320.

Nyman JS, Roy A, Shen X, Acuna RL, Tyler JH, Wang X, 2006. The influence of water removal on the strength and toughness of cortical bone. *J Biomech* 39:931–938.

Oliveira JMQ, de Moura MFSF, Morais JJL, Silva MAL, 2007. Numerical analysis of the MMB test for mixed-mode I/II wood fracture. *Compos Sci Technol* 67:1764–1771.

Olvera D, Zimmermann EA, Ritchie RO, 2012. Mixed-mode toughness of human cortical bone containing a longitudinal crack in far-field compression. *Bone* 50:331–336.

Pallares G, Ponson L, Grimaldi A, George M, Prevot G, Ciccotti M, 2009. Crack opening profile in DCDC specimen. *Int J Fract* 156:11–20.

Palmer LC, Newcomb CJ, Kaltz SR, Spoerke ED, Stupp SI, 2008. Biomimetic systems for hydroxyapatite mineralization inspired by bone and enamel. *Chem Rev* 108:4754–4783.

Parry DA, 1988. The molecular fibrillar structure of collagen and its relationship to the mechanical properties of connective tissue. *Biophys Chem* 29:195–209.

Patil MM, Kulkarni MS, Yerudkar DS, 2020. Determination of elastic properties of bovine femur bone: Solid mechanics approach. *Trends Biomat Artif Organs* 34:67–72.

Pereira B, Xavier J, Pereira F, Morais J, 2018. Identification of transverse elastic properties of the diaphysis of cortical bone. *J Mech Eng Biomechanics* 2:50-55.

Pereira FAM, de Moura MFSF, Dourado N, Morais JJL, Dias MIR, 2014. Bone fracture characterization under mixed-mode I+II loading using the single leg bending test. *Biomech Model Mechanobiol* 13:1331–1339.

Pereira FAM, de Moura MFSF, Dourado N, Morais JJL, Silva FGA, Dias MIR, 2016. Bone fracture characterization under mixed-mode I+II loading using the MMB test. *Eng Fract Mech* 166:151–163.

Pereira FAM, de Moura MFSF, Dourado N, Morais JJL, Xavier J, Dias MIR, 2018. Determination of mode II cohesive law of bovine cortical bone using direct and inverse methods. *Int J Mech Sc* 138–139:448–456.

Pereira FAM, Morais JJL, de Moura MFSF, Dourado N, Dias MIR, 2012. Evaluation of bone cohesive laws using an inverse method applied to the DCB test. *Eng Fract Mech* 96:724–736.

Pereira FAM, Morais JJL, Dourado N, de Moura MFSF, Dias MIR, 2011. Fracture characterization of bone under mode II loading using the end loaded split test. *J Mech Behavior of Biomedical Mater* 4:1764–1773.

Phelps JB, Hubbard GB,Wang X, Agrawal CM, 2000. Microstructural heterogeneity and the fracture toughness of bone. *J Biomed Mater Res* 51:735–741.

Reeder JR, 2003. Refinements to the mixed-mode bending test for delamination toughness. *J Compos Technol Res* 25:191–195.

Reilly DT, Burstein AH, 1975. The elastic and ultimate properties of compact bone tissue. *J Biomech* 8:393–405.

Reilly DT, Burstein AH, Frankel VH, 1974. The elastic modulus for bone. *J Biomech* 7:271–275.

Rho JY, Hobatho MC, Ashman RB, 1995. Relations of mechanical properties to density and CT numbers in human bone. *Med Eng Phys* 17:347–355.

Rho JY, Kuhn-Spearing L, Zioupos P, 1998. Mechanical properties and the hierarchical structure of bone. *Med Eng Phys* 20:92–102.

Rho JY, Tsui, TY, Pharr GM, 1997. Elastic properties of human cortical and trabecular lamellar bone measured by nanoindentation. *Biomaterials* 18:1325–1330.

Ritchie RO, Kinney JH, Kruzic JJ, Nalla RK, 2004. A fracture mechanics and mechanistic approach to the failure of cortical bone. *Fatigue Fract Engng Mater Struct* 28:345–371.

Robinson RA, 1979. Bone tissue: Composition and function. *Johns Hopkins Med J* 145:10–24.

Rosa N, Simoes R, Magalhães FD, Marques AT, 2015. From mechanical stimulus to bone formation: A review. *Med Eng Phys* 37:719–728.

Royce PM, Steinmann B, 2003. *Connective tissue and its heritable disorders: Molecular, genetic, and medical aspects*. John Wiley & Sons. ISBN 978-0-471-46117-3.

Sasaki N, Enyo A, 1995. Viscoelastic properties of bone as a function of water content. *J Biomech* 28:809–815.

Scheiner S, Pivonka P, Hellmich C, 2015. Poromicromechanics reveals that physiological bone strains induce osteocyte-stimulating lacunar pressure. *Biomech Model Mechanobiol* 15:9–28.

Shahar R, Zaslansky P, Barak M, Friesem AA, Currey JD, Weiner S, 2007. Anisotropic Poisson's ratio and compression modulus of cortical bone determined by speckle interferometry. *J Biomech* 40:252–264.

Sharir A, Barak M, Shahar R, 2008. Whole bone mechanics and mechanical testing. *The Veterinary J* 177:8–17.

Sheng W, Ji A, Fang R, He G, ChenC, 2019. Finite element-and design of experiment-derived optimization of screw configurations and a locking plate for internal fixation system. *Comput Math Methods Med* 2019:5636528.

Shore SW, Unnikrishnan GU, Hussein AI, Morgan EF, 2012. Bone biomechanics. In: Winkelstein BA (Ed.), *Orthopaedic biomechanics*. CRC Press, Florida, 3–48.

Shoulders MD, Raines RT, 2009. Collagen structure and stability. *Annu Rev Biochem* 78:929–958.

Skedros JG, Holmes JL, Vajda EG, Bloebaum RD, 2005. Cement lines of secondary osteons in human bone are not mineral-deficient: New data in a historical perspective. *The Anatomical Record Part A* 286A:781–803.

Sousa SDO, 2018. Identificação inversa do módulo de elasticidade longitudinal do tecido ósseo cortical de modelos animais: Ratos sprague dawley e wistar. Master Thesis, UTAD.

Stecco C, Hammer WI, 2015. *Functional atlas of the human fascial system*. Churchill Livingstone, Edinburgh, Ed. ISBN 978-0-7020-4430-4.

Sun L, Fan Y, Li D, Zhao F, Xie T, Yang X, Gu Z, 2009. Evaluation of the mechanical properties of rat bone under simulated microgravity using nanoindentation. *Acta Biomaterialia* 5:3506–3511.

Tang T, Ebacher V, Cripton P, Guy P, McKay H, Wang R, 2015. Shear deformation and fracture of human cortical bone. *Bone* 71:25–35.

Tattersall HG, Tappin G, 1996. The work of fracture and its measurement in metals, ceramics and other materials. *J Mater Sc* 1:296–301.

Timoshenko S, Goodier JN, 1951. *Theory of elasticity*. McGraw-Hill Book Company, New York.

Traub W, Arad T, Weiner S, 1989. Three-dimensional ordered distribution of crystals in turkey tendon collagen fibers. *Proc Natl Acad Sci USA* 86:9822–9826.

Tsai SW, Wu EM, 1971. A general theory of strength of anisotropic materials. *J Comp Mat* 5:58–80.

Turner CH, Burr DB, 1993. Basic biomechanical measurements of bone: A tutorial. *Bone* 14:595–608.

Turner CH, Burr DB, 2001. *Experimental techniques for bone mechanics*. Chapter 7 of Bone Mechanics Handbook, (2nd Edition). Edited by SC Cowin. CRC Press.

Turner CH, Wang T, Burr DB, 2001. Shear strength and fatigue properties of human cortical bone determined from pure shear tests. *Calcif Tissue Int* 69:373–378.

Tzaphlidou M, 2008. Bone architecture: Collagen structure and calcium/phosphorus maps. *J Biol Phys* 34:39–49.

Uda Y, Azab E, Sun N, Shi C, Pajevic PD, 2017. Osteocyte mechanobiology. *Curr Osteoporos Rep* 15:318–325.

Ural A, Vashishth D, 2006. Cohesive finite element modelling of age-related toughness loss in human cortical bone. *J Biomech* 39:2974–2982.

Vanputte C, Russo A, Seeley R, Regan J, 2020. *Seeley's anatomy & physiology*, Twelfth edition. McGraw-Hill Education, New York.

Vashishth D, 2007. Hierarchy of bone microdamage at multiple length scales. *Int J Fatigue* 29:1024–1033.

Vashishth D, Tanner KE, Bonfield W, 1997. Crack growth resistance in cortical bone: Concept of microcrack toughening. *J Biomech* 30:763–769.

Vashishth D, Tanner KE, Bonfield W, 2000. Contribution, development and morphology of microcracking in cortical bone during crack propagation. *J Biomech* 33:1169–1174.

Vashishth D, Tanner KE, Bonfield W, 2001. Fatigue of cortical bone under combined axial–torsional loading. *J Orthop Res* 19:414–420.

Viguet-Carrin X, Garnero P, Delmas PD, 2006. The role of collagen in bone strength. *Osteoporos Int* 17:319–336.

Villarreal XC, Mann KG, Long GL, 1989. Structure of human osteonectin based upon analysis of cDNA and genomic sequences. *Biochemistry* 28:6483–6491.

Wang X, Bank RA, TeKoppele JM, Hubbard GB, Athanasiou KA, Agrawal CM, 2000. Effect of collagen denaturation on the toughness of bone. *Clin Orthop Relat Res* 371:228–239.

Wang XD, Masilamani NS, Mabrey JD, Alder ME, Agrawal CM, 1998. Changes in the fracture toughness of bone may not be reflected in its mineral density, porosity, and tensile properties. *Bone* 23:67–72.

Warshaw J, Bromae TG, Terranova CJ, Enlow DH, 2017. Collagen fiber orientation in primate long bones. *Anat Rec* 300:1189–1207.

Weiner S, Wagner HD, 1998. The material bone: Structure-mechanical function relations. *Annu Rev Mater Sci* 28:271–98.

Xavier J, Garrido N, Oliveira M, Morais J, Camanho P, Pierron F, 2004. A comparison between the Iosipescu and off-axis shear test methods for the characterization of *Pinus Pinaster Ait. Comp Part A* 35:827–840.

Xavier J, Morais J, Pereira F, 2018. Non-linear shear behaviour of bovine cortical bone by coupling the Arcan test with digital image correlation. *Optics and Lasers in Eng* 110:462–470.

Yadav RN, Uniyal P, Sihota P, Kumar S, Dhiman V, Goni V, Sahni D, Bhadada SK, Kumar N, 2021. Effect of ageing on microstructure and fracture behavior of cortical bone as determined by experiment and extended finite element method (XFEM). *Med Eng Phys* 93:100–112.

Yamashita J, Furman BR, Rawls HR, Wang X, Agrawal CM, 2000. The use of dynamic mechanical analysis to assess the viscoelastic properties of human cortical bone. *J Biomed Mater Res* 58:47–53.

Yan J, Mecholsky JrJJ, Clifton KB, Reep RL, 2006. Fracture toughness of manatee rib and bovine femur using a chevron-notched beam test. *J Biomech* 39:1066–1074.

Yang QD, Cox BN, Nalla RK, Ritchie RO, 2006. Re-evaluating the toughness of human cortical bone. *Bone* 38:878–887.

Yeni YN, Brown CU, Wang Z, Norman TL, 1997. The influence of bone morphology on fracture toughness of the human femur and tibia. *Bone* 21:453–459.

Yeni YN, Norman TL, 2000. Calculation of porosity and osteonal cement line effects on the effective fracture toughness of cortical bone in longitudinal crack growth. *J Biomed Mat Research Part B: App Biomater* 51:504–509.

Zhou JJ, Zhao M, Liu D, Liu HY, Du CF, 2017. Biomechanical property of a newly designed assembly locking compression plate: three-dimensional finite element analysis. *J Healthc Eng* 2017:590251.

Zimmermann EA, Launey ME, Barth HD, Ritchie RO, 2009. Mixed-mode fracture of human cortical bone. *Biomater* 30:5877–5884.

Zimmermann EA, Launey ME, Ritchie RO, 2010. The significance of crack-resistance curves to the mixed-mode fracture toughness of human cortical bone. *Biomater* 31:5297–5305.

Zioupos P, 1998. Recent developments in the study of failure of solid biomaterials and bone: Fracture and pre-fracture toughness. *Mater Sc & Eng C* 6:33–40.

Zioupos P, Currey JC, 1998. Changes in the stiffness, strength, and toughness of human cortical bone with age. *Bone* 22:57–66.

Zioupos P, Currey JC, Hamer AJ, 1999. The role of collagen in the declining mechanical properties of ageing human cortical bone. *J Biomedical Mater Res Part A* 45:108–116.

Zioupos P, Wang XT, Currey JD, 1996. Experimental and theoretical quantification of the development of damage in fatigue tests of bone and antler. *J Biomechanics* 29:989–1002.

Zysset PK, 2009. Indentation of bone tissue: A short review. *Osteoporos Int* 20:1049–1055.

Index

Printed in the United States
by Baker & Taylor Publisher Services

Printed in the United States
by Baker & Taylor Publisher Services